ADVANCES IN
HEALTH ECONOMICS AND
HEALTH SERVICES RESEARCH

Volume 7 • 1987

MERGERS IN HEALTH CARE:
THE PERFORMANCE OF
MULTI-INSTITUTIONAL ORGANIZATIONS

ADVANCES IN
HEALTH ECONOMICS AND
HEALTH SERVICES RESEARCH

A Research Annual

MERGERS IN HEALTH CARE:
THE PERFORMANCE OF
MULTI-INSTITUTIONAL ORGANIZATIONS

Editors: RICHARD M. SCHEFFLER
             Department of Social and
             Administrative Health Sciences
             School of Public Health
             University of California, Berkeley

             LOUIS F. ROSSITER
             Department of Health Administration
             Medical College of Virginia
             Virginia Commonwealth University

VOLUME 7 • 1987

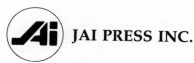 JAI PRESS INC.

Greenwich, Connecticut   *London, England*

CONTENTS

PART II.   BEHAVIOR AND PERFORMANCE

PART III.   ANTITRUST ISSUES

PART IV.   SUMMARY AND REFLECTIONS

LIST OF CONTRIBUTORS

Jeffrey Alexander

Department of Health Services
Administration
University of Alabama,
Birmingham

Gerard Anderson

Center for Hospital Finance and
Management
Johns Hopkins University

Ronald Anderson

Center for Health Administrative
Studies
University of Chicago

Diana Barrett

Center for Health Policy and
Management
Harvard University

James Begun

Department of Health
Administration
Medical College of Virginia

Judith Bentkover

Center for Health Policy and
Management
JFK School of Government
Harvard University

Roger Blair

Public Policy Research Center
University of Florida

David Blumenthal

Center for Health Policy and
Management
JFK School of Government
Harvard University

Paul Campbell

Center for Health Policy and Management
Harvard University

James Carman

Department of Social and Administrative Health Sciences
University of California, Berkeley

Jon B. Christianson

Division of Health Services Research and Policy
University of Minnesota

William Custer

Center for Health Policy Research
American Medical Association

Alan Dobson

Office of Research Health Care Financing Administration

Dan Ermann

Research and Health Care Technology Assessment
National Center for Health Services

James Fesmire

Department of Economics
University of Tampa

Bernard Friedman

Center for Health Services and Policy Research
Northwestern University

Ted Frech, III

Department of Economics
University of California, Santa Barbara

Susan Hughes

School of Medicine
Northwestern University

Philip Jacobs

Department of Economics
University of South Carolina

T. Alan Jensen

Department of Health Administration
Medical College of Virginia

Roice Luke

Department of Health
Administration
Medical College of Virginia

Michael Morrisey

Department of Health Care
Organization and Policy
University of Alabama,
Birmingham

Ellen Morrison

J. L. Kellogg Graduate School of
Management
Northwestern University

Ross Mullner

Center for Health Services
Research
School of Public Health
University of Illinois, Chicago

Robert Musacchio

Center for Health Policy Research
American Medical Association

Catherine Russe

Center for Hospital Finance and
Management
Johns Hopkins University

Mark Schlesinger

Center for Health Policy and
Management
JFK School of Government
Harvard University

Stephen Shortell

J. L. Kellogg Graduate School of
Management
Northwestern University

Frank Sloan

Health Policy Center
Institute for Public Policy Studies
Vanderbilt University

David Starkweather

Department of Social and
Administrative Health Science
University of California, Berkeley

Joseph Valvona   Health Policy Center
                                   Institute for Public Policy Studies
                                   Vanderbilt University

Joan Vitek   J. L. Kellogg Graduate School of
                                   Management
                                   Northwestern University

Lora H. Warner   Department of Health
                                   Administration
                                   Medical College of Virginia

Janet Willer   Center for Health Policy and
                                   Management
                                   American Medical Association

Ronald Wilder   Department of Economics
                                   University of South Carolina

Allan Woodward   Coopers and Lybrand

CONFERENCE PROGRAM COMMITTEE

Gail R. Wilensky
Program Chairman

Vice President
Division of Health Affairs
Project HOPE
Millwood, Virginia

Richard M. Scheffler

Professor
School of Public Health
School of Public Policy
University of California
Berkeley, California

Nelda D. McCall

Director Health Policy Research
SRI International
Menlo Park, California

Louis F. Rossiter

Associate Professor
Department of Health
Administration
Medical College of Virginia
Richmond, Virginia

PREFACE

The Invitational Conference on "Mergers in Health Care: The Performance of Multi-Institutional Organization," was held on Project Hope campus, Millwood, Virginia, on April 9–11, 1986. This conference, second in the series being supported by Project Hope, the University of California, Berkeley, SRI International, and the Medical College of Virginia, produced a series of papers that will become an important benchmark for work in this area. The papers were divided into three major subject areas: Organization and Financing, Behavior and Performance, and Antitrust.

In the session on Organization and Financing, the paper by Shortell et al. looked at the organizational forms of multi-institutional hospital systems and their differences in the types of services provided, cost and indications of quality. Using aggregate data from the American Hospital Association, Muller and Anderson provided an in-depth account of financial ratios for hospitals pre- and post-merger, during the 1980–85 period. Also, utilizing aggregate and national data from the American Hospital Association, the paper by Morrissey and Alexander empirically models some of the important characteristics of hospitals that relate to merger activity. The final paper in this session by Sloan et al., examines the crucial impact that capital has on the growth of multihospital systems, again using aggregate American Hospital Association data.

The second session on Behavior and Performance of Multi-Institutional Health Care Systems began with the Schlesinger et al. paper on access, an often overlooked aspect of multihospital systems. Graduate medical education and its impact on the cost of hospital care has been the focus of attention in the health policy area since the beginning of the Medicare and Medicaid programs. In their paper, Russe and Anderson analyze the difference in the medical education provided by hospitals in investor hospitals after they are purchased as part of a multihospital system.

The next two papers use a case study approach. One is on the Hospital Corporation of America (HCA) and the other is on hospitals in a small area in Northern California. The Barrett and Campbell paper gives us some insight into the internal workings of a major for-profit hospital chain and its approach to, and the problems resulting from, acquisition and mergers. The case studies of individual hospitals were in environments that range in the degree of the competitiveness of the health care market in which they are located. The response to the competitive environments for different hospital organizations form the basis of the Starkweather and Carman paper. The final paper in this session by Begun puzzles over the strategies and behavioral patterns of small multiinstitutional health organizations with respect to their merger activity.

Antitrust is certainly a major ingredient of the environment in which hospital care mergers and acquisitions must function and respond to in order to be successful. Crucial differences between the antitrust treatment of nonprofits as compared to for-profit hospital mergers is explored in the Blair and Fesmire paper. Antitrust in the health care mergers area depends, to a large extent, on market definitions and how the concentration of health care firms in a market is empirically measured. The Jacobs and Wilder paper explores these issues and their implications in crisp detail.

A detailed summary and insightful collection of thoughts on the meaning and significance of papers presented at the conference is provided by Dobson. He and the conference participants were surprised to learn how rapidly the area of mergers and acquisitions in health care has been moving. There was also a clear sense that things are sorting out in this area and that the pace is somewhat slower and more deliberate. Mistakes can be quite costly. Mergers and acquisitions in health care without careful and thoughtful strategies can produce undesired results as windfall market gains disappear. It seems that the rush-in phase for market share is over and that future mergers and acquisitions in health care will be at a slower pace and on firmer economic ground that those observed in the last decade.

Richard M. Scheffler
Louis F. Rossiter
Series Editors

PART I:

ORGANIZATION AND FINANCING

DIVERSIFICATION OF HEALTH CARE SERVICES:

THE EFFECTS OF OWNERSHIP, ENVIRONMENT, AND STRATEGY

Stephen M. Shortell, Ellen M. Morrison, Susan L. Hughes, Bernard S. Friedman, and Joan L. Vitek

I. INTRODUCTION

A major health care trend is the provision of services outside the hospital. Some of these involve services that were traditionally provided as acute inpatient services (for example, surgery and rehabilitation services) while others involved totally new services (for example, sports medicine clinics, and health promotion programs). The need for hospitals to provide more cost-effective inpatient care and develop additional sources of revenue are behind this trend. These in turn are driven by new forms of prospective payment, increased market competition, a surplus of physicians in many specialties, new noninvasive technologies, and changing consumer/ employer expectations (Moxley and Roeder, 1984). The trend involves a major move from acute inpatient delivery of services to a more diversified and vertically integrated health care system involving a wide range of ambulatory care, long-term care, geriatric care, health promotion, and related services.

The primary goal of this paper is to develop and test a model of the factors associated with the provision of diversified services by selected

Advances in Health Economics and Health Services Research, Vol. 7, pgs. 3–40.
Copyright © 1987 by JAI Press Inc.
All rights of reproduction in any form reserved.
ISBN: 0-89232-573-9

multihospital systems and market area comparison hospitals. In addition to the number and type of services offered, data were collected on the provision of charity care and the profitability of each service. Charity care was defined to exclude bad debts and contractual allowances. Profitability was defined as the excess of operating revenues over operating expenses, taking into account both direct and indirect costs. A complete list of services and standard definitions is provided in Appendix A. As shown, these comprise a wide range of over 30 services involving ambulatory care, long-term care, geriatric services, health promotion, diagnostic testing, and alternative delivery systems. A list of 18 unprofitable services as reported by 50% or more of the responding hospitals is presented in Apprendix B.[1]

The model developed argues that diversification is largely a function of environmental factors; hospital ownership, system affiliation and related characteristics; and hospital strategies. Each of these factors have potentially important managerial as well as public policy implications. For example, while some environmental variables such as the sociodemographic characteristics of communities cannot be easily changed by public policy, others such as Medicaid eligibility and payment levels are susceptible to change. In regard to ownership, the continued consolidation of the industry into multiunit systems and affiliations (Ermann and Gabel, 1984) is likely to have important effects on the development and implementation of new programs and services as well as public policies. Of particular significance is the growing role played by investor-owned hospital systems and concern that they may not provide unprofitable services or requisite amounts of charity care (Institute of Medicine, 1986). The underlying strategies pursued by hospitals represents an important and underdeveloped area of inquiry (Shortell et al., 1985a). A greater understanding of the strategies which hospitals pursue will assist policymakers and others in anticipating responses which organizations make to changes in their environment.

Among the questions addressed are the following: (1) Is the number of diversified services offered primarily a function of the environment, hospital ownership form, or the underlying strategies which are pursued? (2) Do Medicaid eligibility and payment levels influence the provision of such services? (3) What role is played by competition and regulation? (4) Do hospitals which belong to systems provide more or fewer such services than freestanding hospitals? (5) Are there differences by ownership form—for example, investor-owned hospitals vs. not-for-profit hospitals? (6) Do sole community hospitals provide more or fewer such services? (7) What factors influence the provision of unprofitable services? (8) What factors explain differences in the provision of charity care?

The major concepts, variables, and measures are developed in the following section. This section is followed by a description of the population studied, the findings, and discussion of the implications for current public and managerial policy.

II. CONCEPTS, VARIABLES, HYPOTHESIS DEVELOPMENT, AND MEASURES

A. Diversification

Diversification is defined as the provision of services which do not involve acute inpatient care. These usually involve the development of new services for new markets. Examples include ambulatory surgery centers, urgent care centers, home health programs, geriatic day care, and health promotion programs. Data for such services were obtained for the most recent fiscal year (in most cases 1984) from a pretested, standardized "Scope of Services" questionnaire (see Appendix A). Information obtained included whether or not the service was offered, the year it was first provided, whether the service was discontinued or in a planning stage, the method by which the service was provided (for example, independently by the hospital, or through a shared service arrangement with another corporation of the same parent organization, or whether it was provided independently by another corporate unit of the same parent organization), number of patient encounters or procedures, approximate percentage of charity care provided as previously defined, and whether or not the service was profitable in regard to operating revenues exceeding operating costs for the period involved. In the absence of strong theoretical reasons for weighting each service, diversification is measured by the additive sum of services offered. Previous research has indicated that such unit weighting schemes are as good or superior to weighted measures (Einhorn and Hogarth, 1975).

B. Environment

The importance of taking into account the environment in which organitzations function is well documented in the organizational (Lawrence and Lorch, 1969; Aldrich, 1979; Meyer, 1978) and health services literature (Starkweather and Cook, 1983). In the present study three sets of environmental variables are considered: the demand for and supply of services in the area, the competitive environment, and the regulatory environment.

C. Demand and Supply

The likely demand for diversified services was measured by median income adjusted by the area wage index, percentage of white-collar and health professional employees, median years of schooling for those 25 and over, births per 1000 population, percentage of the population over 65, and Medicaid eligibility and payment levels. Medicaid eligibility was measured by the percentage of those individuals below the poverty line who were eligible for Medicaid benefits. Medicaid payment generosity was measured by payments per recipient of hospital inpatient and outpatient benefits divided by the state average of hospital expenses per adjusted patient-day. Alternative suppliers of outpatient services was measured by the number of physicians per 1000 population.

Income, education, employment status, the birth rate, and the percentage of the population over 65 are each expected to be associated with greater demand for services. In particular, better-educated higher-income consumers in white-collar and health professions are likely to be more aware of the availability of the new forms of health services and become users. Communities experiencing higher birth rates and a higher percentage of elderly are also more likely to see increased demand for such services. More generous Medicaid eligibility levels provide more people with resources to seek care (Kirkman-Liff, 1985), while higher payment levels encourage hospitals to provide such services. The prediction regarding the physician-to-population ratio is ambiguous. On the one hand, a higher physician-to-population ratio suggests greater opportunities for hospitals and physicians to develop joint ventures involving diversified services. On the other hand, it can be argued that the greater the physician supply, the less need there is for hospitals to provide diversified services. It is suggested that the former effect will dominate, particularly given the increased pressure on hospitals to contain costs by developing a broad range of ambulatory and long-term care services outside the acute inpatient setting. We expect this to be true even where a high number of physicians exist resulting in potential competition between hospitals and physicians for provision of such services.

D.   Competition

Competition is measured by the number of competing hospitals in the study hospital service area, whether or not a competing ambulatory surgery center or urgent care center existed in the hospital's market area, and the Herfindahl Index indicating the percentage concentration of hospital beds in a given study hospital's market area. Determination of competing hospitals was based on work by Luft and Maerki (1984) in which all hospitals within 15 miles of the study hospitals were identified. Most of the study hospitals were then asked to add or eliminate hospitals from this list based on who their competitors really were. Hospitals in markets with two or more competitors were classified as having a relatively high degree of competition (representing the upper 50% of the distribution) and those with only one or no competitors as having a relatively low degree of competition.[2]

Standard economic theory suggests that more goods/services will be provided in more competitive than less competitive markets. Thus, we expect competition to exert a positive influence on the number of diversified services provided.

E. Regulation

The presence of state rate-setting programs and planning agencies which review major capital expenditures may inhibit or promote the growth of alternative services. Separate overall measures of rate review and certificate of need were based on factor analysis of specific components of rate review and certificate of need (Chapko et al. 1984) used in previous research (Shortell et al., 1985c). The specific dimensions included the scope of regulatory activity, stringency of review, degree of enforcement, dollar value of threshold limits, and the length of time that the regulation had been in existence. It is expected that a greater degree of regulation in terms of rate review and certificate of need will be associated with a greater level of alternative services provided as hospitals seek ways to reduce inpatient costs by developing lower-cost out-of-hospital services. Further, it is expected that regulation will narrow any differences found between investor-owned system hospitals and voluntary not-for-profit system hospitals in the provision of charity care. This is because many rate review and certificate-of-need laws require some degree of charity care or provide incentives for such provision (Intergovernmental Health Policy Project, 1984).

F. Hospital Ownership and Related Characteristics

A major issue is the extent to which hospital ownership influences services provision. Hospitals which belong to systems may be able through innovation and experimentation to accelerate the trend toward vertical diversification. Economies of scale and management support functions such as market research and analysis and management information systems development may also provide system hospitals with a competitive advantage over their freestanding counterparts. Thus, other things equal, we expect hospitals belonging to systems to provide a greater number of diversified services than freestanding hospitals.

A related question of interest is whether hospitals belonging to investor-owned systems provide more or fewer such services than hospitals belonging to voluntary not-for-profit systems. Given the growing number of medically indigent and disadvantaged (R. W. Johnson Foundation, 1983; Wilensky and Berk, 1985), the ability and willingness of hospitals to provide needed primary care is an important issue. This is particularly true in regard to unprofitable services. Economic theory suggests that for-profit organizations will not provide unprofitable services (Bays, 1983; Sloan, 1986; Estelle, 1982; Weisbrod, 1977; Hansmann, 1980; Bener, 1983; Preston, 1984), and therefore a major reason for the existence of not-for-profit and public organizations in market economies is to provide such services. Because there is some evidence to support this argument in other industries (Preston, 1984), many are concerned that investor-owned hospitals will not provide unprofitable services. This may result in communities either going without needed care where other providers do not exist or placing a disproportionate burden on voluntary or public hospitals in those communities.

There are few studies to date which address this issue, and the evidence is mixed. Sloan and Vraciu (1983) found that investor-owned hospitals were less likely to provide premature nurseries (which are typically associated with a high percentage of nonpaying patients) but that they were also less likely to provide such profitable services as open-heart surgery, cardiac catheterization, and computerized tomography (CT) scanning. Using American Hospital Association (AHA) data, a recent Institute of Medicine report (1986) found that, controlling for bed size, investor-owned hospitals were less likely to provide outpatient services but were more likely to provide social services and related "community-oriented" services. For contrast, for mental hospitals Schlesinger and Dorwart (1984) found that for-profit providers devoted fewer staff resources to patient care and offered fewer services with community-wide benefits. Without question, most of the burden for uncompensated care has fallen upon the public hospitals (Halmer et al., 1984; Teder, et al., 1984). The question that emerges is whether this will continue as care moves more toward the provision of out-of hospital services.

Ownership categories in the present analysis include being a member of an investor-owned system study hospital, a member of another investor-owned system hospital, a member of a voluntary not-for-profit system study hospital, a member of another voluntary not-for-profit system hospital, voluntary freestanding hospital, and public hospital. There is no basis in economic theory to suggest that one form of ownership will necessarily provide more services than another. Rather, insights are gained from examination of organization goals and the variety of constituents or "stakeholders" in the organization's environment. It is argued that voluntary hospitals have traditionally broader missions and goals than investor-owned hospitals and that they have a more diverse group of constituents than is true of most investor-owned hospitals. Therefore, it is expected that other things being equal voluntary system hospitals will provide more diversified services than investor-owned system hospitals. Unlike the more focused claim of stockholders for dividends and long-term growth in earnings per share, community groups are likely to make multiple and conflicting demands upon the non-investor-owned hospital, reflecting the diverse interests of the community being served.

In regard to the provision of unprofitable services and charity care, it is expected that investor-owned system hospitals will be less likely to provide such care.[3] This is due *only partly* to the discipline of Wall Street and desires of stockholders since given current emphasis on cost containment and market place pressure, all hospitals, including voluntary not-for-profit hospitals, have strong incentives to achieve positive operating margins. A more telling reason is that the constituents of voluntary hospitals are more likely to demand the provision of certain services whether or not they are profitable and hence come to expect the provision of some amount of charity care. Further, some voluntary hospitals, particularly those with a strong religious affiliation, view the provision of some degree of unprofitable services and charity care as an important part of their mission.

Other hospital variables examined include location (central-city urban, non-central-city urban, collar county, nonmetropolitan/rural), number of inpatient services provided, case mix, the number of years the hospital has belonged to a system (for system hospitals only), and whether or not the hospital is the only hospital in the community [that is, sole community provider (Farley, 1985)]. Other things equal, we expect hospitals located in the central-city area to provide more services, reflecting population density and the greater variety of health care needs of inner-city residents. For the latter reason, we also expect hospitals located in the inner-city area to provide more services that are unprofitable and more services for which charity care is offered.

Inpatient services and case mix are each expected to be positively associated with a greater number of diversified services being offered. Diversified alternative services are seen as complimentary to inpatient services, not a substitute for them. For example, the development of an ambulatory surgery center does not result in deletion of a hospital's inpatient surgery unit. In regard to case mix, the more severe a hospital's given patient mix, the greater the cost containment pressures and the greater the incentive to develop an array of diversified services to which patients can be discharged as soon as possible. In addition, pressures on inpatient profit margins provide incentives for hospitals to develop profitable diversified service lines.

It is expected that the longer a hospital has belonged to a system, the more likely it is to provide a greater number of services as it gains experience in utilizing corporate staff and resources. We also expect that being a sole community provider will narrow differences between investor-owned and voluntary system hospitals in regard to services offered, unprofitable services offered, and charity care. This is because sole community provider status increases the importance to the investor-owned hospital of providing needed community services given the lack of available alternatives.

G. Strategy and Structure

The link between hospital ownership characteristics and the environment in which hospitals function is the strategies which hospitals develop to influence the environment. Strategy is defined as the plans and activities developed by an organization in pursuit of its goals and objectives, particularly in regard to positioning itself to meet external environmental demands relative to its competition (Shortell et al., 1985b). Under cost-based reimbursement, there was relatively little incentive for hospitals to think or act strategically. We argue that such behavior was just beginning to emerge at the time that the diversification data were collected (coinciding with the introduction of Medicaid Prospective Payment in 1983/84) and therefore do not expect strong effects of strategy at this time. The strategy variables are included to capture possible initial effects and suggest future relationships.

We are interested in the overall strategic direction of hospitals as well as more specific product-service/market strategies. Based on Miles and Snow (1978) and Hambrick (1983), we measure the overall strategic orientation of hospitals in regard to four categories: prospector, analyzer, defender, and reactor. A *prospector* organization is one which is consistently first in providing a new product or service. It consistently attempts to pioneer. An *analyzer* is an organization which is seldom first in providing a new product or service but which, by carefully analyzing the market and what others are doing, will often enter later and attempt to provide the service better or somewhat differently (that is, create a market niche) than the early entrants. The *defender* is an organization that offers a relatively stable set of products and services. It tends to ignore changes that have no direct impact on current areas of operation and concentrates instead on doing the best job possible in its own area. A *reactor* organization doesn't have a consistent pattern. Sometimes it is an early entrant into a new market, sometimes it will wait until others have entered, and sometimes it will not do anything unless forced by external pressures. Perceptions of each hospital's overall strategic orientation were obtained from each hospital's chief executive officer. In general we expected that hospitals characterized as prospectors or analyzers would provide more diversified services than those characterized as defenders or reactors because prospectors and analyzers have a more active orientation toward the marketplace.

The extent to which hospitals explicitly undertake diversification strategies was measured by the degree of emphasis given by chief executive officers to new product/service development and new market development for 15 specific services.[4] These services ranged from inpatient surgical care to health promotion programs. It was expected that hospitals which were more aggressively pursuing such diversification strategies would be more likely to provide a greater number of out-of-hospital services.

Based in part on the work of the Boston Consulting Group (Henderson, 1973), we also measured each hospital's overall product/service portfolio. Data were obtained for each of the 15 services previously noted regarding their perceived market share, market growth potential, and profitability. Market share was defined as (1) more than 1.5 times that of our closest competitor; (2) up to 1.5 times that of our closest competitor; (3) about the same as our closest competitor; (4) less than 1.5 times that of our closest competitor; or (5) more than 1.5 times less than our closest competitor. Market growth potential was measured by the following categories: (1) no growth—service may actually be declining; (2) 1–10% growth in volume per year; (3) 11–50% growth in volume per year; and (4) greater than 50% growth in volume per year. Profitability was measured by the following three categories: (1) unprofitable; (2) operating revenues exceed operating expenses by 1–10% per year; and (3) operating revenues exceed operating expenses by greater than 10% per year.

These data were factor-analyzed (see Appendix C) to derive an overall measure of each hospital's product/service portfolio. In general, the greater degree to which the portfolio emphasized high market share services, the more likely the hospital was expected to provide a higher number of diversified services and conversely for a low share portfolio.

We also took into account centralization of decision making by measuring each hospital's chief executive officer's perception of the level at which 12 pretested standardized decisions were made. Examples of such decisions included (1) choosing a marketing plan for a new outpatient service at an individual hospital; (2) deciding to involve more physicians in individual hospital governance; (3) acquiring a new hospital; and (4) deciding to add an ambulatory surgery center at an individual hospital. Decision-making levels were ordered from 1 (low) to 6 (high) and included levels below the individual hospital chief executive officer, the hospital chief executive officer, individual hospital board, divisional or regional management, corporate management, and corporate board. It was expected that the greater the degree to which decision making was decentralized, the greater the number of alternative services which would be offered because decentralization provides better ability to adopt to local market conditions and service demands.

III. METHODS

The "Scope of Services" questionnaire was sent to 574 hospitals belonging to eight multiunit systems located in different areas of the country. The systems were selected as part of a larger study of the strategies, structure, and performance of multiunit hospital systems based on ownership, size, geographic location, differences in centralization of decision making, and related factors. Three of the systems were investor-owned and five were voluntary not-for-profit systems. Completed questionnaires were received from 96% (n = 550) of the system hospitals. In addition, questionnaires were sent to 853 competing hospitals operating in the same market area as the system hospitals or, in the case of sole community hospitals, matched on bed size and location within the same state. Completed questionnaires were received from 66% (n = 564) of the comparison hospitals.

There were no differences between respondents and nonrespondents in regard to bed size, occupancy rates, or degree of teaching involvement. Respondents were somewhat more likely to be located in the South Atlantic region of the country and somewhat less likely to be located in the Pacific region. Respondents were also more likely to be investor-owned and somewhat less likely to be not-for-profit secular or Catholic hospitals. Finally, a somewhat lower percentage of respondents were located in the central-city urban area, and somewhat more respondents than nonrespondents were located in nonmetropolitan rural areas.

The equations took the following general functional form:

$$SOS = F(SD_V, C_V, R_V, HO_V, S_V) + e_i,$$

where
SOS	=	number of diversified services provided;
SD_V	=	vector of sociodemographic demand and supply variables;
C_V	=	vector of competition variables;
R_V	=	vector or regulation variables;
HO_V	=	vector of hospital ownership variables and related characteristics;
S_V	=	vector of strategy and structure variables;
e_i	=	error term.

Each vector or set of variables was forced into the equation in the order indicated. Table 1 summarizes the means and standard deviations for each of the variables along with the predicted relationship to the dependent variables of interest. Except for a correlation of .67 between bed size and number of inpatient services provided and .57 between bed size and case mix, multi-collinearity is largely absent.

Table 1. Descriptive Statistics on Analytical Variables

Variable	Data Source	Mean[a] (Standard Deviation)	Predicted Relationship to Dependent Variable		
			Total Services Offered	Unprofitable Services Offered	Charity Care
Diversification					
Number of Alternative Services Offered—**CTTOTA**	Scope of Services Questionnaire	9.69 (4.91)			
Number of Unprofitable Services Offered—**LOSSCTA**	Scope of Services Questionnaire	1.78 (2.05)			
Percent of Services for Which Some Charity Care is Provided—**CHARY**	Scope of Services Questionnaire	75% (37.02)			
Environment					
1. *Demand and Supply*					
Median Income Adjusted by Area Wage Index— **MFINCADJ**	Area Resource File	20,411.33 (6,937.02)	+	–	–
Percent White Collar and Percent Health Professionals— **EMPLMIX**	Area Resource File	60.07 (39.68)	+	–	–
Median Years of Schooling For Those Over 25—**YRSSCH25**	Area Resource File	11.77 (.70)	+	–	–
Births Per 1,000 Population— **BIRTHSPT**	Area Resource File	16.76 (3.88)	+	?	?
Percent of Population Over 65— **PCTOV65**	Area Resource File	11.76 (4.34)	+	–	–

(*continued*)

Table 1. (continued)

Variable	Data Source	Mean[a] (Standard Deviation)	Predicted Relationship to Dependent Variable		
			Total Services Offered	Unprofitable Services Offered	Charity Care
Medicaid Eligibility Levels— **MCELIG**	Area Resource File	.49 (.25)	+	−	−
Medicaid Payment Levels— **MCPMT**	Area Resource File	2.09 (.62)	+	−	−
Physicians Per 1000 Population— **ACTMDSPT**	Area Resource File	.68 (1.08)	?	?	?
2. *Competition*					
Number of Competing Hospitals in Hospital's Service Area— **COMPA:** High = 2 Plus Low = 1 or None	Luft and Maerki Tape	.61 (.48)	+	+	+
Presence of a Competing Ambulatory Surgery Center or Urgent Care Center— **COMPB**	Questionnaire	.22 (.41)	+	+	+
Herfindahl Index of Concentration— **HRTI005**	Luft and Maerki Tape	.42 (.42)	?	?	?

Table 1. (continued)

Variable	Data Source	Mean[a] (Standard Deviation)	Predicted Relationship to Dependent Variable		
			Total Services Offered	Unprofitable Services Offered	Charity Care
3. Regulation					
Overall Rate Review Measure— **REVIEW**	Univ. of Washington Regulation Study	−2.36 (8.20)	+	+	+
Overall Certificate-of-Need measure—**CON**	Univ. of Washington Regulation Study	−1.94 (4.49)	?	?	+
Interaction of Hospital Competition and Regulation— **RRCOMPA**	Luft and Maerki Tape & Univ. of Washington Study	−1.11 (6.61)	+	+	+
Interaction of Ambulatory Care Competition & Regulation— **RRCOMPB**	Questionnaire & Univ. of Washington Study	−.454 (3.88)	+	+	+
Hospital Ownership and Related Characteristics					
Ownership					
Study Investor-Owned System— **IOSYS**	Questionnaire and AHA Tape	.43 (.49)	+	−	−
Study Not For Profit System– **NFPSYS**		.07 (.25)	+ +	+	+
Non-Study Investor-Owned System—**IOSYSN**		.04 (.21)	+	−	−
Non-Study Not for Profit System— **NFPSYSN**		.09 (.29)	+ +	+	+

(*continued*)

Table 1. (continued)

Variable	Data Source	Mean[a] (Standard Deviation)	Total Services Offered	Unprofitable Services Offered	Charity Care
				Predicted Relationship to Dependent Variable	
Freestanding Not for Profit Hospitals (Omitted Category)—**FSNFP**		.36 (.35)			
Public Hospital— **PUBLIC**		.01 (.09)	+ +	+ +	+ +
Location					
Central City Urban—**URBAN**	Area Resource File	.20 (.40)	+	+	+
Non-Central City (Omitted Category)		.31 (.46)			
Collar County— **COLLAR**		.27 (.44)	?	?	?
Non-Metropolitan Rural—**RURAL**		.22 (.41)	−	+	+
Case mix—**CM84**	HCFA	1.08 (.10)	+	?	?
Number of Inpatient Services Provided— **AHATOT**	AHA Tape	23.85 (9.95)	+	?	?
Number of Years in System—**SYSTEM**	Questionnaire	7.28 (6.66)	+	−	−
Sole Community Provider— **DUMMY18**	Luft and Maerki and AHA Tape	.21 (.40)	−	+	+
Bedsize—**BEDS**	AHA Tape	204 (179.59)	+	+	?
Strategy and Structure (for System Hospitals Only)					
Overall Strategic Orientation	Strategy Questionnaires				
Prospector— **PROSP**		.22 (.416)	+	+	?
Analyzer— **ANALY**		.63 (.484)	+	+	?

Table 1.   (continued)

Variable	Data Source	Mean[a] (Standard Deviation)	Predicted Relationship to Dependent Variable		
			Total Services Offered	Unprofitable Services Offered	Charity Care
Defender (Omitted Category)		.02 (.139)			
Reactor—**REACT**		.118 (.323)	+	?	?
New Product/New Market Development Score—**NSMDEV**	Strategy Questionnaires	40.48 (16.08)	+	+	?
High Market Share Score—**HISHARE**	Strategy Questionnaires	.730 (.995)	+	−	−
Low Market Share Score—**LOSHARE**	Strategy Questionnaires	.956 (.871)	−	+	+
Centralization of Decision Making—**DSCORE**	Decision-Making Questionnaire	3.45 (.46)	−	+	?

Note: [a] The means and standard deviations are for the pooled sample involving both study system hospitals and their market area comparison hospitals, except for the strategy and structure variables which apply to the system hospitals only. + + Particularly strong positive relationship.

IV.   FINDINGS

A.   Number of Diversified Services Provided

As shown in Table 2, the number of services provided is most strongly associated with hospital characteristics and sociodemographic demand and supply variables. As predicted, not-for-profit system hospitals provide more alternative services than freestanding not-for-profit hospitals, although there is no significant difference for the investor-owned system hospitals. Larger size hospitals, hospitals located in the central-city and hospitals with a more severe case mix also provide more diversified services, as predicted. The number of inpatient services provided is also strongly associated with provision of a greater number of alternative services.

As predicted, Medicaid payment and, in particular, eligibility levels are positively associated with the number of alternative services provided, as is education. Contrary to prediction, rate-review intensity is negatively associated with provision of alternative services. The number of competing

Table 2. Number of Alternative Services Offered: Least Squares
Results for Overall Population[a]
(System and Comparison Hospitals, N = 1029)

Variable	Unstandardized Coefficient (Std. Error)	T Value	Standardized Coefficient
ACTMDSPT	.213 (.168)	1.271	.047
BIRTHSPT	−.060 (.047)	−1.279	−.047
MCPMT	.422* (.242)	1.741	.054
MFINCADJ	−.000 (.000)	.380	.011
EMPLMIX	.002 (.004)	.512	.014
MCELIG	2.118*** (.615)	3.442	.110
YRSSCH25	.430** (.216)	1.994	.062
PCTOV65	−.023 (.039)	−.584	−.020
CON	−.006 (.033)	−.187	−.006
REVIEW	−.039** (.020)	−1.968	−.065
HRTI005	.121 (.349)	.346	.010
COMPB	.381 (.347)	1.099	.032
COMPA	.433 (.403)	1.074	.043
PUBLIC	.727 (1.426)	.510	.014
NFPSYSN	.513 (.491)	1.046	.030
IOSYSN	.119 (.673)	.177	.005
COLLAR	.410 (.396)	1.036	.037

Table 2.   (continued)

Variable	Unstandardized Coefficient (Std. Error)	T Value	Standardized Coefficient
NFPSYS	1.790** (.595)	3.008	.093
AHATOT	.103*** (.019)	5.457	.210
IOSYS	−.206 (.323)	−.637	−.021
CENTRAL	.832** (.414)	2.009	.067
CM84	4.558** (1.66)	2.753	.099
RURAL	.498 (.451)	1.104	.042
DUMMY18	.113 (.461)	.245	.009
BEDS	.005*** (.001)	3.985	.174
(CONSTANT)	−6.040 (2.978)	−2.028	—

Notes: [a]Adjusted R^2 = .28; F = 16.83; $P \leq .001$.
   * $P \leq .10$.
  ** $P \leq .05$.
 *** $P \leq .001$.

hospitals and presence of an ambulatory surgery/urgent care center are each positively associated with provision of more alternative services, but are not statistically significant.

The findings for the system-owned hospitals incorporating the strategy and structure variables are shown in Table 3. Again, the sociodemographic and hospital characteristics explain the greatest percentage of the variation in the number of diversified services provided. After all other variables were entered into the equation, the strategy/structure variables explained an additional two percent of the variation.

As shown, there is no significant difference between investor-owned system hospitals and not-for-profit system hospitals, once the other variables are taken into account. Of particular note is that, as predicted, hospitals with a high percentage of low market share services (LOSHARE)

Table 3. Number of Alternative Services Offered: Least Squares
Results for *System Hospitals Only*[a]
(N = 306)

Variable	Unstandardized Coefficient (Std. Error)	T Value	Standardized Coefficient
ACTMDSPT	.430 (.355)	1.212	.087
BIRTHSPT	.060 (.091)	.658	.054
MCPMT	.243 (.552)	.441	.028
MFINCADJ	.000 (.000)	.577	.032
EMPLMIX	.002 (.007)	.265	.014
MCELIG	.861 (1.188)	.725	.049
YRSSCH25	.024 (.429)	.055	.003
PCTOV65	−.038 (.072)	−.525	−.038
CON	−.130* (.076)	−1.723	−.106
REVIEW	−.038 (.045)	−.830	−.056
HRTI005	.257 (.665)	.386	.024
COMPB	−.051 (.602)	−.084	−.005
COMPA	1.915** (.736)	2.602	.198
AHATOT	.083** (.034)	2.435	.146
SYSMEM	.044 (.038)	1.178	.063

Table 3. (continued)

Variable	Unstandardized Coefficient (Std. Error)	T Value	Standardized Coefficient
COLLAR	1.101 (.738)	1.492	.105
IOSYS	−.790 (.876)	−.902	−.060
CM84	2.406 (3.452)	.697	.046
CENTRAL	1.863** (.741)	2.516	.166
STATBD	.008** .003	2.647	.187
RURAL	.617 (.833)	.740	.052
DUMMY18	1.319 (1.019)	1.295	.106
REACT	1.690 (1.516)	1.115	.117
NSMDEV	−.007 (.015)	−.493	−.026
HISHARE	−.617 (.379)	−1.627	−.131
DSCORE	1.040* (.565)	1.840	.104
PROSP	1.795 (1.459)	1.230	.160
LOSHARE	−.891** (.442)	−2.015	−.166
ANALY	1.363 (1.358)	1.004	.141
(CONSTANT)	−5.453 (6.492)	−.840	—

Notes: [a]Adjusted R^2 = .24; F = 4.34; $P \leq .0001$.
  * $P \leq .10$.
 ** $P \leq .05$.
*** $P \leq .001$.

offer fewer diversified services regardless of ownership. Also, as predicted, hospitals characterized as prospectors, analyzers, and reactors offer more services than defenders, although the findings are not statistically significant. Contrary to expectation there is some suggestion that centralization of decision-making is positively associated with provision of a greater number of alternative services. Bed size, central-city location, and number of inpatient services are each positively associated as well.

For the system hospitals sample, neither Medicaid payment nor Medicare eligibility levels remain significant. What appears to be more important is certificate-of-need intensity and the number of competing hospitals. Certificate-of-need intensity has a negative effect on the number of diversified services provided, while the number of competing hospitals has a positive effect.

B. Number of Unprofitable Services Provided

Table 4 presents the results pertaining to the number of unprofitable alternative services provided. Again, sociodemographic variables and hospital characteristics account for most of the variation. Not-for-profit system hospitals offer significantly more unprofitable alternative services than not-for-profit freestanding hospitals, while investor-owned system hospitals offer fewer. As before, bed size, central-city location, and number of inpatient services offered are each positively associated with the provision of more unprofitable alternative services.

Contrary to expectation, Medicaid payment and eligibility levels are each positively associated with the number of unprofitable services provided. The birth rate is negatively associated. Neither rate-review intensity, certificate-of-need intensity, nor the competition measures are significantly associated with the number of unprofitable services offered.

In Table 5, the results for the system owned hospitals are presented. While as a group, the inclusion of the strategy/structure variables adds about two percent to the percentage of variation explained, none of the strategy/structure variables by themselves are significant. As shown, investor-owned system hospitals offer significantly fewer unprofitable services than not-for-profit systems hospitals. Again, central-city location, and bed size are positively associated with the provision of unprofitable services. The birth rate, percent of the population over 65, and certificate-of-need intensity are each negatively associated with the provision of unprofitable services.

C. Percent of Services for Which Charity Care is Offered

For the pooled sample, Table 6 presents the results regarding charity care. As shown, investor-owned system hospitals provide significantly

Table 4. Number of *Unprofitable* Alternative Services Offered: Least Squares Results for all Hospitals[a]
(N = 1029)

Variable	Unstandardized Coefficient (Std. Error)	T Value	Standardized Coefficient
ACTMDSPT	.041 (.074)	.550	.022
BIRTHSPT	− .066*** (.021)	− 3.149	− .124
MCPMT	.280** (.107)	2.606	.085
MFINCADJ	− .000 (.000)	− .148	− .004
EMPLMIX	− .000 (.001)	− .087	− .003
MCELIG	1.031*** (.273)	3.778	.128
YRSSCH25	.109 (.095)	1.140	.037
PCTOV65	− .026 (.018)	− 1.464	− .054
CON	− .002 (.0148)	− .148	− .005
REVIEW	− .007 (.009)	− .767	− .027
HRTI005	.119 (.155)	.767	.025
COMPB	− .041 (.154)	− .265	− .008
COMPA	.035 (.179)	.196	.008
AHATOT	.083*** (.034)	2.435	.146
PUBLIC	.920 (.633)	1.454	.042
NFPSYSN	.240 (.218)	1.103	.034
IOSYSN	− .217 (.298)	− .729	− .023

(*continued*)

Table 4. (continued)

Variable	Unstandardized Coefficient (Std. Error)	T Value	Standardized Coefficient
COLLAR	.160 (.175)	.914	.035
NFPSYS	1.149*** (.264)	4.354	.143
AHATOT	.027*** (.008)	3.195	.131
IOSYS	− .281*** (.143)	− 1.961	− .068
CENTRAL	.482** (.184)	2.624	.093
CM84	.748 (.734)	1.018	.039
RURAL	.230 (.200)	1.147	.047
DUMMY18	− .182 (.205)	− .891	− .036
BEDS	.002** (.000)	3.097	.144
(CONSTANT)	− 1.241 (1.321)	− .940	—

Notes: ªAdjusted R^2 = .18; F = 10.21; P ≤ .0001.
  * P ≤ .10.
 ** P ≤ .05.
*** P ≤ .001.

fewer services involving charity care than do not-for-profit freestanding hospitals. Hospitals located in rural areas also provide significantly fewer services involving charity care than do hospitals located in non-central-city urban areas. As expected, Medicaid eligibility level and education are negatively associated with the percentage of services involving charity care. Both certificate-of-need and rate-review intensity have positive significant associations as expected, while the number of competing hospitals is negatively associated with the percentage of services for which charity care is provided.

Finally, Table 7 shows the charity care results for the study system hospitals only. As shown, there is no significant difference between investor-owned system hospitals and not-for-profit *system* hospitals in the percentage of services for which charity care is provided. The

Table 5. Number of *Unprofitable* Alternative Services Offered: Least Squares Results for *System Hospitals Only*[a]
(N = 306)

Variable	Unstandardized Coefficient (Std. Error)	T Value	Standardized Coefficient
ACTMDSPT	.102 (.147)	.693	.051
BIRTHSPT	−.084** (.038)	−2.237	−.190
MCPMT	.089 (.229)	.389	.025
MFINCADJ	−.000 (.000)	−.280	−.016
EMPLMIX	.001 (.003)	−.217	−.012
MCELIG	.429 (.494)	.870	.060
YRSSCH25	−.131 (.178)	−.737	−.045
PCTOV65	−.068** (.030)	−2.265	−.170
CON	−.089** (.031)	−2.826	−.178
REVIEW	−.019 (.019)	−1.033	−.072
HRTI005	.182 (.276)	.660	.042
COMPB	.095 (.250)	.380	.022
COMPA	.177 (.306)	.577	.045
AHATOT	.018 (.014)	1.239	.076
SYSMEM	.009 (.016)	.593	.033
COLLAR	.417 (.307)	1.360	.098
IOSYS	−1.352*** (.364)	−3.712	−.253

(*continued*)

Table 5.   (continued)

Variable	Unstandardized Coefficient (Std. Error)	T Value	Standardized Coefficient
CM84	.476 (1.434)	.332	.023
CENTRAL	1.010*** (.308)	3.283	.222
STATBD	.004** (.001)	2.858	.208
RURAL	.218 (.346)	.630	.046
DUMMY18	.243 (.423)	.574	.048
REACT	.361 (.630)	.574	.062
NSNDEV	−.004 (.006)	−.701	−.038
HISHARE	−.132 (.158)	−.835	−.069
DSCORE	.244 (.235)	1.037	.060
PROSP	.852 (.606)	1.405	.187
LOSHARE	−.154 (.184)	−.838	−.071
ANALY	.799 (.564)	1.416	.204
(CONSTANT)	2.382 (2.698)	.883	—

Notes: [a]Adjusted R^2 = .20; F = 3.62; $P \leq .0001$.
 * $P \leq .10$.
 ** $P \leq .05$.
 *** $P \leq .001$.

strategy/structure variables as a set exert relatively little influence. The variable which comes closest to approaching significance is HISHARE, representing hospitals which have a high percentage of services involving high market share. Such hospitals tend to provide more services involving charity care.

Table 6. Percent of Alternative Services for which *Charity Care* is
Provided: Least Squares Results for all Hospitals
(N = 846)

Variable	Unstandardized Coefficient (Std. Error)	T Value	Standardized Coefficient
ACTMDSPT	−1.085 (1.547)	−.702	−.032
BIRTHSPT	−.363 (.447)	−.812	−.038
MCPMT	−2.702 (2.498)	−1.082	−.043
MFINCADJ	−.000 (.000)	−.885	−.031
EMPLMIX	−.025 (.031)	−.803	−.029
MCELIG	−16.014** (5.846)	−2.739	−.112
YRSSCH25	−5.673** (2.057)	−2.755	−.107
PCTOV65	−.525 (.373)	−1.407	−.062
CON	.561* (.319)	1.757	.068
REVIEW	.343* (.190)	1.802	.076
HRTI005	2.299 (3.358)	.685	.027
COMPB	2.941 (3.295)	.892	.033
COMPA	−7.101* (3.908)	−1.817	−.093
NFPSYSN	2.494 (4.849)	.514	.019
IOSYSN	6.479 (6.962)	.931	.034
PUBLIC	1.432 (16.613)	.086	.003
COLLAR	−3.942 (3.752)	−1.051	−.047

(continued)

Table 6. (continued)

Variable	Unstandardized Coefficient (Std. Error)	T Value	Standardized Coefficient
NFPSYS	−5.340 (5.600)	−.954	−.038
AHATOT	.200 (.184)	1.084	.052
CENTRAL	−3.998 (3.923)	−1.019	−.043
IOSYS	13.300*** (3.123)	−4.254	−.179
CM84	−5.999 (15.688)	−.382	−.017
RURAL	−8.398** (4.290)	−1.957	.094
DUMMY18	−.051 (4.502)	−.011	−.000
BEDS	.011 (.011)	.980	.053
(CONSTANT)	185.239 (28.658)	6.464	—

Notes: ᵃAdjusted R^2 = .05; F = 2.93; P ≤ .0001.
  * P ≤ .10.
  ** P ≤ .05.
  *** P ≤ .001.

The differences which emerge are related primarily to location, case mix, and competition. System hospitals located in collar-county or rural areas provide fewer services involving charity care than do those located in non-central-city urban areas. Case mix is negatively associated with the provision of services involving charity care. The presence of a competing ambulatory surgery/urgent care center is positively associated with the provision of services involving charity care. Finally, the greater the percentage of white-collar and health professionals in the labor force, the fewer the percentage of services provided involving charity care. The regulatory variables involving certificate-of-need intensity and rate-review intensity, which were significant in the pooled sample, are also positive in the system hospital only equation, but are not significant.

Table 7. Percent of Alternative Services for which *Charity Care* is Provided: Least Squares Results for *Systems Hospitals* Only[a] (N = 281)

Variable	Unstandardized Coefficient (Std. Error)	T Value	Standardized Coefficient
ACTMDSPT	−1.659 (3.763)	−.441	−.037
BIRTHSPT	.667 (.889)	.750	.072
MCPMT	−3.883 (5.345)	−.727	−.052
MFINCADJ	−.000 (.000)	−1.237	−.080
EMPLMIX	−.121* (.071)	−1.719	−.109
YRSSCH25	−3.940 (4.254)	−.926	−.064
MCELIG	−2.898 (11.702)	−.248	−.019
PCTOV65	−.769 (.709)	−1.085	−.091
CON	.458 (.738)	.621	.044
REVIEW	.494 (.451)	1.094	.087
HRTI005	7.331 (6.580)	1.114	.080
COMPB	11.124** (6.060)	1.836	.120
COMPA	−15.273** (7.449)	−2.050	−.185
AHATOT	.136 (.340)	.399	.028
SYSMEM	−.436 (.373)	−1.169	−.074
COLLAR	−14.446** (7.254)	−1.991	−.162
IOSYS	−.956 (8.786)	−.109	−.008

(continued)

Table 7. (continued)

Variable	Unstandardized Coefficient (Std. Error)	T Value	Standardized Coefficient
CENTRAL	−11.425 (7.406)	−1.543	−.118
CM84	−84.950** (35.409)	−2.399	−.187
RURAL	−17.319** (8.265)	−2.096	−.171
STATBD	.039 (.031)	1.265	.104
DUMMY18	−1.457 (10.219)	−.143	−.014
REACT	3.901 (15.086)	.259	.032
NSMDEV	−.029 (.149)	−.195	−.012
PROSP	−1.419 (14.484)	−.098	−.015
HISHARE	5.833 (3.771)	1.547	.147
DSCORE	.245 (5.590)	.044	.003
LOSHARE	4.173 (4.387)	.951	.091
ANALY	−1.472 (13.590)	−.108	−.018
(CONSTANT)	233.168 (64.346)	3.624	—

Notes: [a]Adjusted R^2 = .05; F = 1.57; P ≤ .036.
   * P ≤ .10.
   ** P ≤ .05.
   *** P ≤ .001.

V.   DISCUSSION AND IMPLICATIONS

The findings which emerge shed some light on the questions raised in the introductory section of the paper. The main implications are elaborated below.

A. Provision of Diversified Alternative Services

Not-for-profit system hospitals are more active in providing diversified alternative services than their freestanding counterparts. Not-for-profit system hospitals also provide more such services than investor-owned system hospitals, but the difference is not statistically significant once other factors are taken into account. Among those factors is the overall service portfolio which hospitals offer. System hospitals which have a high percentage of services with low market share are less likely to offer a high number of diversified alternative services. An inability to capture higher market share may limit a hospital's ability to provide a more diversified service mix. This is particularly true when low market share is also combined with low market growth potential, resulting in a cash drain which limits the ability to develop a broad array of services.

As expected, bed size and central-city location are associated with greater alternative services provision, as is the number of inpatient services offered. The latter suggests that inpatient services and alternative out-of-hospital services are not a substitute for each other in terms of their presence or absence, but rather a complement or supplement. Such services may, of course, substitute for each other in regard to volume, as in the case of selected surgical procedures which are done increasingly on an ambulatory rather than an inpatient basis. The positive effect of case mix on the number of alternative services provided suggests that such services are needed to support early discharge policies involving the need for a continuum of follow-up care in the community. This finding is particularly important to the extent that hospitals continue to attract sicker patients.

The positive effects of Medicaid payment and eligibility level suggests that hospitals, both investor-owned and not-for-profit, are responsive to state policies. Increasing eligibility levels means that more medically indigent people will have at least some coverage for care, making it more attractive to hospitals to develop new services. Higher payment levels, of course, add to the incentive. To the extent that such services result in lower cost alternatives to inpatient utilization, the overall policy effect may be positive. However, as noted earlier, the present findings indicate a positive association between the number of inpatient services provided and the number of alternative services provided, although this relationship is not specific to Medicaid nor does it consider actual volume of services rendered.

None of the competition measures were significant in the pooled sample. However, among the system hospitals there is some evidence that the number of competing hospitals has a positive effect on the number of alternative services provided. The effect of competition on diversification requires continued study. It is possible that both the number of new services started and the number of services dropped will be highest where competition is the greatest. The net effect may be a slight increase in the overall number of services provided in more competitive markets versus less competitive markets. The finding in regard to centralization of decision making being associated with provision of a greater volume of alternative services may reflect the fact that corporate office sets overall strategic direction for the provision of such services. Support for this was found in extensive corporate office interviews conducted with top executives from each system. Thus, even though implementation and choice may be left up to each hospital, the overall decision to become involved in ambulatory surgery, long-term care, health promotion, and related activities may be set centrally. This will be explored further in ongoing research.

Finally, the negative associations of rate review intensity on alternative services provision are puzzling. It was expected that as pressure is put on hospitals' inpatient rates, incentives are created for developing lower cost outpatient and alternative service options. Yet we find a net effect of fewer such services provided the greater the degree of rate review intensity.

B. The Provision of Unprofitable Services

The results clearly indicate that investor-owned system hospitals provide fewer unprofitable services than other hospital ownership forms. These results are consistent with economic theory (Bays, 1983; Sloan, 1986; Estelle, 1982; Weisbrod, 1977; Hansmann, 1980; Bener, 1983; Preston, 1984). In addition, bed size, number of inpatient services and central-city location are positively associated with the provision of more unprofitable services. Central-city urban hospitals serving a higher percentage of the medically indigent, may be less able to generate profits from alternative services which when combined with decreasing inpatient profit margins, may make these hospitals particularly vulnerable financially.

It was originally felt that higher Medicaid payment and eligibility levels would be associated with fewer unprofitable services provided. However, the fact that both have positive significant signs suggests that hospitals are more willing to provide services which are usually unprofitable when eligibility and payment levels are high. This is because the higher levels help to assure that the operating deficits for these services may decline in the long run. This, of course, will depend on the scope of benefits covered by the Medicaid program.

C. Provision of Charity Care

Investor-owned system hospitals offer a lower percentage of services for which charity care is provided than not-for-profit freestanding hospitals. However, when considering *system* hospitals only, no significant difference emerges in the provision of charity care between investor-owned *system* hospitals and not-for-profit *system* hospitals. These findings indicate the importance of considering both *system* and *ownership* effects.

Again, Medicaid policies are important. High Medicaid eligibility levels are associated with fewer services for which charity care is provided. In brief, the more people which are included in the Medicaid program, the less is the need for hospitals to offer as much charity care assuming that care for these people was previously totally uncompensated.

The positive effects of certificate-of-need and rate-review intensity on the percentage of services for which charity care is provided indicate the potential importance of state level policies on hospital provision of charity care. Such policies, however, do not address the issue of the ongoing ability of hospitals to provide such care. The larger issue, of course, is the need to finance a predetermined level of benefits for the medically indigent. Hospitals, whether they be investor-owned or not-for-profit, are only one player in the solution.

Finally, it is important to note that the provision of charity care appears to be particularly problematic for hospitals located in rural areas and hospitals in highly competitive markets. Both are associated with fewer services for which charity care is provided.

VI. SUMMARY

The present findings suggest that the trend toward greater diversification of hospital services is likely to be most strongly influenced by state Medicaid policies and certain hospital characteristics. Increasing Medicaid eligibility and payment levels is likely to have a positive effect on services diversification. Growth in the number of inpatient services provided and a more severe case mix are also likely to be involved with greater service diversification. Affiliation with a not-for-profit hospital system is likely to be associated with more diversified hospital services but not affiliation with an investor-owned system. There is also some indication that the overall portfolio of services which a hospital offers in regard to market share and market growth characteristics influences diversification. Specifically, a low market share portfolio is likely to be associated with less diversification. Competition is likely to be associated with more diversification; particularly for hospitals belonging to systems. The effect of competition on hospital strategy and services diversification is a particularly important area for further investigation.

Increasing Medicaid payment and eligibility levels are also likely to have a positive effect on the provision of services which are usually unprofitable. Raising such levels is likely to be particularly beneficial to inner-city hospitals who are already providing a greater number of such services. However, the present data suggest that investor-owned hospitals are least likely to provide such services.

Increasing Medicaid eligibility levels is also likely to be associated with fewer services for which charity care has to be provided. State regulation in the form of rate review and certificate of need is likely to be associated with more services for which hospitals provide some charity care. But such policies alone do not deal with the larger issue of how to finance care for the medically indigent. Present data suggest the charity care issue may be particularly salient in markets characterized by a relatively high degree of competition. Finally, investor-owned hospitals provide as many services involving charity care as not-for-profit system hospitals, although investor-owned system hospitals provide fewer such services than not-for-profit freestanding hospitals.

Throughout, the findings indicate the importance of distinguishing between *ownership* and *system* affiliation. Previous research has failed to make a distinction between ownership form and system affiliation, thus attributing to ownership form differences which, as present findings suggest, appear to be more associated with system affiliation.

Underlying hospital strategies have relatively little influence on diversification at present. However, it is expected that they will be more strongly associated with such behavior in future years as cost containment and competitive pressures force hospitals to shift from an operational orientation to a more strategic orientation.

The present findings will be explored further in ongoing research; in particular, in examining changes in strategies and diversification of services over time. Such analysis will also examine the effects of diversification on the cost and quality of care provided for both investor-owned and not-for-profit system hospitals.

APPENDIX A:
SCOPE OF SERVICES—
LIST AND DEFINITIONS

1. Ambulatory Care

Ambulatory surgery: One-day surgical care performed on an outpatient basis. The patient is discharged 1 to 3 hours after surgery when recovery from anesthesia is complete.

Chemotherapy/radiation therapy: Services of chemical and radiation treatment provided on an outpatient basis to oncology patients.

Crisis intervention: Services including telephone "hot line" numbers and specialized medical, counseling, or legal services aimed at delivering service to persons at a time of crisis.

Kidney dialysis: The provision of renal dialysis on an outpatient basis.

Outpatient psychiatric/mental health services: Services which include counseling, therapy, prescription of medication, medication evaluations, and psychiatric day care to persons with psychological problems.

Rehabilitation program: Services which include coordinated restorative services for physical, occupational, speech, and other disorders.

Sports medicine and/or orthopedic clinic: Outpatient health care services designed for the prevention and treatment of athletic injuries and disorders of the skeletal system.

Substance abuse program: Provision of medical and/or social services designed to mitigate or reverse the effects of drug and/or alcohol abuse and to reduce or eliminate abuse. This includes individual counseling and therapy, group counseling, detox, and Antabuse.

Urgent care/immediate care center(s):   A facility or program designed to provide health care to people who do not have a serious disease or injury.

Women's health services: Provision of routine gynecological care, birth control and family planning, prenatal care, and problem pregnancy referral and counseling.

2.   Geriatric Care

Assessment/consultation/case management program: Services which include comprehensive assessment of a geriatric patient's functional level, medical condition, and mental, emotional, social, and financial status. *Note:* This service may be provided on an inpatient or outpatient basis.

Day care: Centers providing health, recreation, and social services to older adults; include intake assessment, health monitoring, occupational therapy, personal care, a noon meal, and transportation.

Home-delivered meals: Provision of meals on a daily basis to homebound older adults who are not able to prepare meals for themselves.

3.   Health Promotion

Health screening: Services designed to identify certain conditions or diseases—e.g., diabetes, hypertension—in the absence of a recognizable symptom or to identify persons who may be susceptible to a given condition or disease.

Immunizations: Inoculations provided to children and adults to immunize them against common infectious diseases—e.g., measles, diphtheria, whooping cough.

Occupational health: Health care services directed toward persons exposed to a particular environmental or physical hazard because of their occupation.

School health exams: Physical exams, including early preventive, screening, and detection programs, provided to students.

Wellness programs: Provision of health status evaluation or lifestyle modification courses—e.g., smoking cessation, weight control, hypertension.

4.   Home Health Care/Extended Care

Durable medical equipment/medical supplies: Provision of beds, infusion pumps, walkers, wheelchairs, IV medication supplies, etc. to patients at home due to illness, injury, impairment, or advanced age.

Hospice: Services provided to patients with terminal illness. These services may be provided solely in the home or in combination with inpatient or outpatient programs.

Infusion therapy: Provision and care of intravenous lines for chemotherapy, enteral or parenteral nutrition, antibiotics, etc. to patients at home.

Physical therapy: Provision of coordinated, physical restorative services to patients at home.

Respiratory care: Provision of personal assistance and services to ventilator and respirator-dependent persons at home.

Skilled nursing: Provision of intermittent nursing care to patients who require primarily convalescent, rehabilitative, and/or restorative services.

5.   Outpatient Diagnostic Services

CT Scan: Computerized axial tomography equipment used as a diagnostic tool.

Hematology/biochemistry laboratory: Chemical and cellular analysis of blood provided on an outpatient basis.

NMR or MRI: Nuclear magnetic resonance, magnetic resonance imaging, etc. used as diagnostic tools.

Radiology: Diagnostic laboratory providing X-ray and related services on an outpatient basis.

Ultrasound: Sound wave equipment used as a diagnostic tool.

6.   Service Delivery Alternatives

HMO: Staff, group, network, or independent practice association model health maintenance organization sponsored in whole or in part by the hospital.

Hospital-sponsored primary care group practice: Group practices of three or more physicians designed to provided comprehensive primary care to patients under a contractual relationship with the hospital.

PPO/PPA: Preferred provider organization/preferred provider arrangement sponsored in whole or in part by the hospital or for which the hospital is a preferred provider.

APPENDIX B: UNPROFITABLE SERVICES LIST

Crisis Intervention
Outpatient Psychiatric/Mental Health Services
Urgent Care/Immediate Care Centers
Geriatric Assessment/Consultation/Case Management Program
Geriatric Day Care
Home-Delivered Meals to the Elderly
Health Screening Services
Immunization Services
Occupational Health Services
School Health Exams
Wellness Programs
Disease/Condition-Specific Counseling and Education
Community Health Lectures, Classes, and Health Fairs
Family Planning and Preparation: Parenting and Sibling Education
Hospice
Swing Bed
Intermediate Care/Skilled Nursing Facility
Hospital-Sponsored Primary Care Group Practice

APPENDIX C:
SERVICE PORTFOLIO FACTOR ANALYSIS

Table C-1. Principal Components Analysis with Varimax Rotation[a]

	Factor 1 Loadings (High Share)	Factor 2 Loadings (Low Share)
"STARS"	.815	.11
"CASH COWS"	.814	− .086
"WILDCATS"	.048	.792
"DOGS"	− .026	.760

	Percent Variance Explained
Factor 1 Eigenvalue = 1.34	33.6%
Factor 2 Eigenvalue = 1.21	30.3%

STARS   = high market share, high market growth potential services

CASH COWS = high market share, low market growth potential services

WILDCATS = low market share, high market growth potential services

DOGS   = low market share and low market growth potential services

---

Note: (1) Each hospital's percentage of the 15 services which fell into each of the cells was multiplied by the factor score coefficient and summed to form a high share and low share measure, respectively.

(2) Profitability did not load on either factor and was, therefore, deleted from present analysis.

ACKNOWLEDGMENTS

Support for this research was provided by Grant No. 09181 from the Robert Wood Johnson Foundation, Princeton, New Jersey and Grant No. HS 05159–01 and 02 from the National Center for Health Services Research and Health Care Technology Assessment. Appreciation is expressed to Lee Berg, James Coverdill, Valerie Crum, and Binne Douglas for their assistance in data-processing analysis and manuscript preparation. Appreciation is also expressed to the Hospital Research and Educational Trust of the American Hospital Association for their endorsement and support of the Scope of Services questionnaire associated with this study. Finally, the comments of Jon Christianson on an earlier draft of this paper are gratefully acknowledged.

NOTES

1.   The 50% criterion for *all institutions* was used rather than each hospital's own experience with unprofitable services in order to recognize that for a given hospital unprofitability may be due to hospital management inefficiency. By selecting only those services for which 50% or more of *all* hospitals reported being unprofitable, greater confidence is gained that these services are more problematic in regard to their inherent profitability.

2.   It is recognized that some two-hospital communities may experience more intense competition between those two hospitals than other communities in which three or more hospitals exist. However, on average, competition is likely to be more intense and complex the greater the number of competing hospitals in a given market area.

3.   One might ask why the investor-owned hospital would provide *any* such care. The answer lies, first, in recognizing that some services which may be unprofitable in terms of accounting costs may still have overall economic benefit to the organization through generating inpatient admissions or referrals to other hospital services. Second, investor-owned hospitals must maintain some degree of legitimacy and credibility with local communities in addition to satisfying Wall Street analysts and current and future investors. Providing some amount of such care is "good business" and an important part of being a responsible corporate citizen.

4.   These services included general inpatient surgical care, general inpatient medical care, general inpatient obstetrics care, general inpatient pediatrics care, general inpatient psychiatric care, outpatient renal dialysis, outpatient diagnostic centers, home health care, long-term care, ambulatory surgery, urgent care centers, inpatient or outpatient rehabilitation, outpatient alcoholism treatment, inpatient alcoholism treatment, and health promotion.

Respondents were asked to allocate 100 points across the following four categories: (1) market penetration; (2) new market development; (3) product refinement; and (4) new product development. *Market penetration* was defined as further penetration of current markets using existing services. *New market development* was defined as providing services to new populations or geographic areas. *Product refinement* was defined as the modification or upgrading of an existing product or service. *New product development* was defined as the development of a product or service not currently offered.

REFERENCES

Aldrich, Howard E. (1979), *Organizations and Environments*. Englewood Cliffs, NJ: Prentice-Hall.

Bays, Carson W. (1983), "Why Most Private Hospitals are Non-Profit." *Journal of Policy Analysis and Management* (February):366–385.

Bener, Avner (1983), "Non-Profit Organizations: Why Do They Exist in Market Economies?" Working Paper No. 51, Program A—Non-Profit Organization, Institution for Social and Policy Studies, Yale University.

Carman, James M., David B. Starkweather, and M. Haley (1985), "Competition, Markets, and Strategy In the Hospital Industry: A Comparison of Three Communities." Western Center for Health Planning and University of California, Berkeley, Western Consortium for the Health Professions Inc., Working Paper, September.

Chapko, Michael, Douglas A. Conrad, Karen S. Cook, et al. (1984), "Development of a Multi-Dimensional Measure of Capital Expenditure and Rate Regulation for Hospitals." Working Paper, Department of Health Services, University of Washington, Seattle.

Einhorn, Hillel J. and Robin M. Hogarth (1975), "Unit Weighting Schemes for Decision-Making." *Decision Science* pp. 171–192.

Ermann, Dan and John Gable (1984), "Multi-Hospital Systems: Issues and Empirical Findings." *Health Affairs* (Spring):50–64.

James, Estelle (1982), "Production, Consumption, and Cross-Subsidization in Non-Profit Organizations." Working Paper No. 30, Program on Non-Profit Organizations, Institution for Social and Policy Studies, Yale University.

Farley, Dean A. (1985), "Sole Community Hospitals: Are They Different?" Hospital Studies Program, National Center for Health Services Research and Development and Health Care Technology Assessment, Rockville, MD.

Feder, Judith, Jack Hadley, and Ross Mullner (1984), "Poor People and Poor Hospitals: Implications for Public Policy." *Journal of Health Politics, Policy and Law* 9(Summer):237–250.

Institute of Medicine (1986), *The For-Profit Health Care Enterprise*, National Academy of Sciences, Washington, DC, June.

Halmer, Carl G., D. D. Bradham, and M. Ruschefsky (1984), "Investor-Owned and Not-For-Profit Hospitals: Beyond the Cost and Revenue Debate." *Health Affairs* pp. 133–136.

Hambrick, Donald C. (1983), "Some Test of the Effectiveness and Functional Attributes of Miles and Snow's Strategic Types." *Academy of Management Journal* 26(March):5–26.

Hansmann, Henry B. (1980), "The Role of Not-For-Profit Enterprise." *Yale Law Journal* 89(5):835–901.

Henderson, Bruce D. (1973), "The Experience Curve Reviewed: IV. The Growth Share Matrix of the Product Portfolio." Boston: The Boston Consulting Group.

Intergovernmental Health Policy Project (1984), "The Status of Major State Policies Affecting Hospital Capital Investment." Washington, D.C., The George Washington University, July, 1984.

Kirkman-Liff, B. (1985) "Refusal of Care: Evidence From Arizona." *Health Affairs* (Winter):15–25.

Lawrence, Paul R. and Jay W. Lorsch (1969), *Organization and Environment: Managing Differentiation and Integration*. Homewood, IL: Irwin.

Luft, Harold S. and Susan C. Maerki (1984), "Competitive Potential of Hospitals and Their Neighbors." *Contemporary Policy Issues* (Winter):89–102.

Meyer, Marshall W. and Associates (1978), *Environments and Organizations*. San Francisco: Jossey Bass.

Miles, Raymond E. and Charles C. Snow (1978), *Organizational Strategy, Structure, and Process.* New York: McGraw-Hill.

Moxley, John H. III, and Penelope C. Roeder (1984), "New Opportunities for Out-of-Hospital Health Services." *New England Journal of Medicine* (January 19):194.

Preston, Ann E. (1984), "The Non-Profit Firm: A Potential Solution to Inherent Market Failures." Working Paper No. 77, Department of Economics, Wellesley College, pp. 1–21.

The Robert Wood Johnson Foundation (1983), *Update Report on Access to Health Care for the American People.* Princeton, NJ.

Schlesinger, Mark and Robert Dorwart (1984), "Ownership and Mental Health Services: A Reappraisal of the Shift Toward Privately Owned Facilities." *New England Journal of Medicine* 311(5):959–965.

Shortell, Stephen M., Ellen M. Morrison, and Shelley Robbins (1985a), "Strategy Making in Health Care Organizations: A Framework and Agenda for Research." *Medical Care Review* 42(2):219–266.

Shortell, Stephen M., Ellen M. Morrison, and Shelley Robbins (1985b), "Strategy Making in Health Care Organizations: A Framework and Agenda for Research." *Medical Care Review* 42(2):220.

Shortell, Stephen M., Michael A. Morrisey, and Douglas A. Conrad (1985c), "Economic Regulation and Hospital Behavior: The Effects on Medical Staff Organization and Hospital–Physician Relationships." *Health Services Research* 20(5):597–628.

Sloan, Frank A. (1986), "Property Rights in the Hospital Industry." In H. E. Frech, III (ed.), *Health Care Policy* (forthcoming).

Sloan, Frank A. and Robert Vracru (1983), "Investor-Owned and Not-For-Profit Hospitals: Addressing Some Issues." *Health Affairs* 2(Spring):25–37.

Starkweather, David and Karen S. Cook (1983), "Organization–Environment Relations." In Stephen M. Shortell and Arnold D. Kaluzny (eds.), *Health Care Management: A Text in Organization Theory and Behavior.* New York: Wiley.

Weisbrod, Burton A. (1977), *The Voluntary Non-Profit Sector: Economic Analysis.* Lexington, MA: Lexington Books.

Wilensky, Gail R. and Mark L. Berk (1985), "The Poor, Sick, Uninsured and the Role of Medicaid." In *Hospitals and the Uninsured Poor: Measuring and Pain for Uncompensated Care.* New York: United Hospital Fund, pp. 33–47.

A DESCRIPTIVE AND FINANCIAL RATIO ANALYSIS OF MERGED AND CONSOLIDATED HOSPITALS:

UNITED STATES, 1980–1985

Ross M. Mullner and Ronald M. Andersen

I. INTRODUCTION

Sieverts and Sigmond predicted in 1970 that the last quarter of this century would be an era in which virtually every health institution in the country would be involved in one or more mergers. This prediction appears to be coming true (Finkler and Horowitz, 1985).

The last several years have witnessed an increase in the number and frequency of hospitals involved in mergers and consolidations. In just the first three months of this year (1986), for example, several significant combinations have occurred or are under discussion. In the San Francisco Bay area, three health institutions (Pacific Presbyterian Medical Center, San Francisco; Marin General Hospital, Greenbrae; and Mills-Peninsula Hospital, San Mateo) completed California's largest merger between independent, not-for-profit hospitals. In Rochester, Minnesota, the Mayo Clinic, St. Mary's Hospital of Rochester, and Rochester Methodist Hospital have agreed to merge. In Chicago, two of the city's largest medical research and teaching institutions—Michael Reese Hospital and Medical Center and the University of Chicago Hospitals and Clinics—have formed a joint com-

Advances in Health Economics and Health Services Research, Vol. 7, pgs. 41–58.
Copyright © 1987 by JAI Press Inc.
ISBN: 0-89232-573-9

mittee of trustees to explore the possibility of merger. This merger would create the Chicago area's largest medical complex. In Baltimore, officials at Johns Hopkins Hospital announced plans to consolidate with three other hospitals (Wyman Park Health System, North Charles General Hospital, and Francis Scott Key Medical Center) and an HMO (the Hopkins Health Plan). In the Boston area, Brookline Hospital is in the process of becoming a subsidiary of the parent company of Beth Israel Hospital.

Despite the increasing number, frequency, and importance of mergers and consolidations in the health care industry, there have been relatively few large scale studies of the phenomena. With the exception of the work of Treat (1972), Starkweather (1981), and Finkler and Horowitz (1985), most of the literature on the topic is primarily concerned with specific individual hospitals involved in a particular merger or consolidation and is highly anecdotal in nature, limited to a small geographic area, and deals with a small period of time. Also, most of the studies were conducted in the late 1960s and 1970s before the beginning of the current period of major health care cost-containment efforts, changes in the financing of hospital care, increased competition from alternative types of health care delivery systems, and precipitous declines in hospital inpatient admissions and lengths of stay.

The objective of this paper is two-fold: first, to describe the institutional, locational, and environmental characteristics of hospitals that combined through merger or consolidation in the United States during the six years 1980–1985; and, second, to examine whether these combinations, in the short term, resulted in significant overall financial changes in the hospitals.

Institutional characteristics to be examined include major types of hospitals, total number of hospital beds, ownership types, and occupancy rates. Locational characteristics include geographic location by U.S. Census Division, whether or not the hospital is located in a metropolitan [Metropolitan Statistical Area (MSA)] or nonmetropolitan (non-MSA) area, and the population size of the area. Environmental characteristics include the percentage of hospital patients (as measured by gross patient revenue) by major payor types (Medicare, Medicaid, Blue Cross/Blue Shield, commercial insurance, self-pay, and other) and whether or not the hospitals are in rate-setting states.

To investigate the overall financial changes resulting from the merger or consolidation, before-and-after comparisons are made. Financial ratio analyses of the overall financial conditions (liquidity and profitability) of hospitals for several years before they merged or consolidated are compared to the financial conditions of the same set of hospitals after they combined. Three ratios are used: the current ratio, the total margin ratio, and the net-to-gross-patient-revenue ratio.

II. METHODS

The definition of a merger and a consolidation used in this study is that of Finkler and Horowitz (1985). Specifically, these terms are defined as follows:

A merger is a type of combination where organization A merges with organization B and the resulting combined entity is organization A. No "new" accounting entity is created. For example, suppose that the local community hospital in Bergen combined with the local community hospital in Essex, the adjoining town, and both facilities remained open. If one of the two hospitals became a legal part of the other, taking on the other hospital's name, it would technically be considered a merger. Thus, if Bergen Community Hospital combined with Essex Community Hospital and the resulting organization was Bergen Community Hospital, this combination would properly be called a merger.

A consolidation is a combination where organization A combines with organization B and the combined entity is organization C. Thus a new entity is created. For example, suppose that a new, not-for-profit corporation, Bergen–Essex Hospitals, was formed and both Bergen Community Hospital and Essex Community Hospital combined as parts of this new Bergen–Essex Hospitals corporation. Such a combination would technically be considered a consolidation.

All data sources used in this study come from the American Hospital Association (AHA). The initial source data on the specific hospitals involved in a merger or a consolidation, and the date of its occurrence, were obtained from the AHA's membership files. These files contain information reported primarily by individual (freestanding) hospitals (for the most part, data on multihospital system mergers and acquisitions are not included) that are registered with (approximately 98% of all U.S. hospitals), and in most cases members of, the association.

Data describing the hospitals' institutional, locational, and environmental characteristics and financial conditions were obtained from the AHA's Annual Surveys of Hospitals. Further, extensive computer editing and checking were used to ensure the accuracy of these data.

Because there may be important differences in the characteristics, types, and outcomes of hospitals that merged vs. those that consolidated, and because these differences may have influenced the decision to enter a specific type of combination, data for hospitals that consolidated or merged were analyzed separately.

Hospitals involved in a merger were divided into those that were acquired and those that were acquiring. In total, 55 hospitals were identified as acquired and 45 as acquiring. Data describing the characteristics of all of these hospitals were obtained for the one-year period prior to their merger.

Hospitals involved in a consolidation were divided into those hospitals that combined, on the one hand, and the new hospitals that resulted, on the other. In total, 62 hospitals were identified as being combined into 32 new hospital entities. Data describing the characteristics of the hospitals that combined were obtained for the one-year period prior to their consolidation. Data on the characteristics of the new hospital entity were obtained for the one-year period after the consolidation.

For comparison purposes, data on all hospitals in the United States were also obtained for the approximate midpoint of the study by pooling the characteristics of all hospitals for 1982/83.

Construction of the tables in this manner, although somewhat procrustean, was necessary for comparison purposes.

III. HOSPITAL CHARACTERISTICS

A. Institutional Characteristics

Table 1 presents data for merged (acquired and acquiring), consolidated (combining and new hospital entity), and all U.S. hospitals, respectively, by major type of hospital—community and specialty. Community hospitals are defined by the AHA as all nonfederal, short-term, general, and other special hospitals, excluding hospital units of institutions, whose facilities and services are available to the public. Specialty hospitals (noncommunity) are defined as including psychiatric hospitals; tuberculosis and other respiratory disease hospitals; federal hospitals; and other special hospitals, for example, mental retardation, rehabilitation, and chronic or long-term disease hospitals.

The table shows that acquiring and consolidating hospitals were likely to be community hospitals. Of hospitals involved in a merger, 91% of the acquiring hospitals were community hospitals. For hospitals involved in a consolidation, the percentages were 92% for combining hospitals and 91% for the resulting new hospital entities. In contrast, specialty hospitals made up a greater proportion than that for the nation of acquired hospitals. Twenty-nine percent of the acquired hospitals were specialty hospitals, while the percentage for all U.S. hospitals was 16%.

The bed sizes of hospitals involved in a merger or consolidation are shown in Table 2. The table shows that the largest percentages of hospitals were in the smallest bed-size category, 6–99 beds, for both acquired hospitals (45%) and combining hospitals (42%). These percentages were very similar to that for all U.S. hospitals (45%). In contrast, acquiring and new hospital entities had a much higher proportion of hospitals in the largest bedsize category, 500+ beds (29% and 28%, respectively) compared to 8% for all U.S. hospitals. Most mergers involved a larger hospital acquiring

Table 1. Type of Hospitals Involved in a Merger or Consolidation, 1980–1985

Hospital Type	Hospitals That Merged		Hospitals That Consolidated		All Hospitals in the United States[a]
	Acquired Hospitals	Acquiring Hospitals	Combining Hospitals	New Hospital Entity	
Community	71%(39)	91%(41)	92%(57)	91%(29)	84%(5,792)
Speciality	29%(16)	9%(4)	8%(5)	9%(3)	16%(1,110)
Total	100%(55)	100%(45)	100%(62)	100%(32)	100%(6,902)

[a]Data were pooled for 1982/83, the two years representing the midpoint of the study.

45

Table 2. Bed Size of Hospitals Involved in a Merger or Consolidation, 1980–1985

Hospital Bed Size	Hospitals That Merged		Hospitals That Consolidated		All Hospitals in the United States
	Acquired Hospitals	Acquiring Hospitals	Combining Hospitals	New Hospital Entity	
6–99	45%(25)	13%(6)	42%(25)	9%(3)	45%(3,091)
100–199	35%(19)	18%(8)	16%(10)	32%(10)	23%(1,584)
200–299	13%(7)	22%(10)	19%(12)	9%(3)	12%(829)
300–399	7%(4)	13%(6)	11%(7)	19%(6)	7%(498)
400–499	0%(0)	5%(2)	6%(4)	3%(1)	5%(337)
500+	0%(0)	29%(13)	6%(4)	28%(9)	8%(563)
Total	100%(55)	100%(45)	100%(62)	100%(32)	100%(6,902)

46

a small-size hospital. For consolidations, a similar pattern also occurred, with a large hospital combining with a small hospital.

Table 3 presents the ownership type of merged and consolidated hospitals. The table shows that, in general, nongovernment not-for-profit hospitals were more likely to be involved in a merger or a consolidation. Seventy-four percent of the acquiring hospitals were nongovernment not-for-profit, as were 74% of the combining and 78% of the new hospital entities. This compares to 51% for all hospitals. Acquired hospitals were similar to all hospitals in terms of their ownership. This means that they were more likely to be government or investor-owned than were acquiring or consolidating hospitals.

The occupancy rate of merged and consolidated hospitals is shown in Table 4. Hospitals that are acquired or are going to combine have occupancy rates similar to the country as a whole. In contrast, acquiring hospitals have high occupancy rates (about one-half had occupancy rates of more than 80% compared to 28% for all hospitals).

B. Locational Characteristics

Table 5 shows the geographic location by U.S. Census Division of merged, consolidated, and all U.S. hospitals. Mergers were more likely to take place in the Middle Atlantic Census Division (37% of the acquired and 31% of the acquiring hospitals compared to only 11% of all hospitals were Middle Atlantic). In contrast, the location of consolidations was more similar to the locations of all hospitals in the country.

Table 6 presents merged, consolidated, and all U.S. hospitals by location in metropolitan (MSA) or nonmetropolitan (non-MSA) areas. A large proportion of mergers, as compared to all hospitals in the nation, were located in metropolitan areas. Seventy-six percent of the acquired and 73% of the acquiring hospitals were located in these areas. In contrast, combining and new hospital entities had very similar proportions to that of all U.S. hospitals. Sixty-one percent of the combining, 59% of the new hospital entities, and 57% of all U.S. hospitals were located in metropolitan areas.

Table 7 shows the sizes of the communities where hospital mergers and consolidations occurred. Merging hospitals were less likely to be in small communities of 1–49,999 inhabitants. For hospitals that merged, 24% of the acquired and 27% of the acquiring hospitals were in this category compared to 43% for the country as a whole. Consolidating hospitals were similar to all hospitals, with 39% of combining hospitals and 41% of the new hospital entities being in the smallest communities.

Generally, both merging and consolidating hospitals are more likely to be in the largest communities. Thus, while 14% of the nation's hospitals are located in communities of 2.5+ million inhabitants, 22% of the ac-

Table 3. Ownership Type of Hospitals Involved in a Merger or Consolidation, 1980–1985

Hospital Ownership Type	Hospitals That Merged		Hospitals That Consolidated		All Hospitals in the United States
	Acquired Hospitals	Acquiring Hospitals	Combining Hospitals	New Hospital Entity	
Nongovernment not-for-profit	55%(30)	74%(33)	74%(46)	78%(25)	51%(3,528)
State & local government	25%(14)	22%(10)	8%(5)	6%(2)	30%(2,088)
Investor-owned	18%(10)	2%(1)	15%(9)	13%(4)	14%(942)
Federal	2%(1)	2%(1)	3%(2)	3%(1)	5%(344)
Total	100%(55)	100%(45)	100%(62)	100%(32)	100%(6,902)

48

Table 4. Occupancy Rate of Hospitals Involved in a Merger or Consolidation, 1980–1985

Hospital Occupancy Rate	Hospitals That Merged		Hospitals That Consolidated		All Hospitals in the United States
	Acquired Hospitals	Acquiring Hospitals	Combining Hospitals	New Hospital Entity	
0–20%	0%(0)	0%(0)	0%(0)	0%(0)	1%(56)
21–40%	13%(7)	5%(2)	5%(3)	0%(0)	7%(476)
41–60%	16%(9)	2%(1)	26%(16)	16%(5)	22%(1,546)
61–80%	44%(24)	44%(20)	48%(30)	53%(17)	42%(2,926)
81–100%	27%(15)	49%(22)	21%(13)	31%(10)	28%(1,898)
Total	100%(55)	100%(45)	100%(62)	100%(32)	100%(6,902)

49

Table 5. Census Division of Hospitals Involved in a Merger or Consolidation, 1980–1985

Hospital Census Division	Hospitals That Merged		Hospitals That Consolidated		All Hospitals in the United States
	Acquired Hospitals	Acquiring Hospitals	Combining Hospitals	New Hospital Entity	
New England	7%(4)	9%(4)	10%(6)	9%(3)	5%(364)
Middle Atlantic	37%(20)	31%(14)	13%(8)	14%(4)	11%(781)
South Atlantic	7%(4)	7%(3)	10%(6)	9%(3)	15%(1,021)
East North Central	15%(8)	16%(7)	19%(12)	19%(6)	16%(1,043)
East South Central	4%(2)	3%(2)	6%(4)	6%(2)	8%(546)
West North Central	7%(4)	9%(4)	6%(4)	9%(3)	13%(892)
West South Central	16%(9)	16%(7)	8%(5)	9%(3)	14%(959)
Mountain	2%(1)	2%(1)	10%(6)	9%(3)	6%(452)
Pacific	5%(3)	7%(3)	18%(11)	16%(5)	12%(844)
Total	100%(55)	100%(45)	100%(62)	100%(32)	100%(6,902)

Table 6. Metropolitan/Nonmetropolitan Status of Hospitals Involved in a Merger or Consolidation, 1980–1985

| Hospital Status | Hospitals That Merged | | Hospitals That Consolidated | | All Hospitals in the United States |
	Acquired Hospitals	Acquiring Hospitals	Combining Hospitals	New Hospital Entity	
Metropolitan	76%(42)	73%(33)	61%(38)	59%(19)	57%(3,908)
Nonmetropolitan	24%(13)	27%(12)	39%(24)	41%(13)	43%(2,994)
Total	100%(55)	100%(45)	100%(62)	100%(32)	100%(6,902)

Table 7. Community Size of Hospitals Involved in a Merger or Consolidation, 1980–1985

Hospital Community Size	Hospitals That Merged		Hospitals That Consolidated		All Hospitals in the United States
	Acquired Hospitals	Acquiring Hospitals	Combining Hospitals	New Hospital Entity	
1–49,999	24%(13)	27%(12)	39%(24)	41%(13)	43%(2,993)
50,000–99,999	5%(3)	2%(1)	0%(0)	0%(0)	1%(74)
100,000–249,999	5%(3)	9%(4)	10%(6)	9%(3)	9%(611)
250,000–499,999	18%(10)	20%(9)	3%(2)	3%(1)	9%(635)
500,000–999,999	15%(8)	13%(6)	6%(4)	6%(2)	10%(680)
1,000,000–2,499,999	11%(6)	13%(6)	19%(12)	22%(7)	14%(963)
2,500,000+	22%(12)	16%(7)	23%(14)	19%(6)	14%(946)
Total	100%(55)	100%(45)	100%(62)	100%(32)	100%(6,902)

quired and 16% of the acquiring hospitals are located in such communities. A similar pattern occurred for hospitals which consolidated. Twenty-three percent of the combining and 19% of the new hospital entities were located in this community size category.

C. *Environmental Characteristics*

Table 8 shows that merging and consolidating hospitals are more often found in rate-setting states than would be expected from the distribution of all U.S. hospitals. While 13% of all U.S. hospitals are in rate-setting states, 34% of the acquired, 29% of the acquiring, 18% of the combining, and 19% of the new hospital entities were in such states.

Table 9 shows the percentage and dollar amount of gross patient revenue by major payer types (Medicare, Medicaid, commercial, Blue Cross/Blue Shield, self-pay, and other) at merged, consolidated, and all U.S. hospitals.

New hospital entities had the largest percentage (42%) of gross patient revenues from Medicare. This percentage was larger than that for all U.S. hospitals (38%). In contrast, acquired hospitals had the lowest percentage (32%).

Acquired hospitals had the largest percentage (13%) of gross patient revenues from Medicaid. This percentage was larger than that for all U.S. hospitals (11%). In contrast, new hospital entities had the lowest percentage (6%).

Merging and consolidating hospitals all had lower percentage revenues from commercial insurance than that for all U.S. hospitals. The percentages were 15% for acquired hospitals, 18% for acquiring hospitals, 19% for combining hospitals, and 14% for new hospital entities, while the figure for all hospitals was 21%.

In contrast, merging and consolidating hospitals all had higher percentages of revenues from Blue Cross/Blue Shield than that for all U.S. hospitals. For all U.S. hospitals the percentage was 16%. For merging hospitals the percentages were 18% for acquired and 26% for acquiring hospitals. For consolidating hospitals the percentages were 17% for combining and 23% for new hospital entities.

The percentages from self-pay were fairly consistent for merging (8% for acquired and 6% for acquiring), consolidating (7% for combining and 7% for new hospital entities), and all U.S. hospitals (8%).

For other, the largest percentages were for acquired (14%) and combining hospitals (11%). The percentage for new hospital entities was 11%. The lowest percentage was for acquiring hospitals (4%). For all U.S. hospitals the percentage was 6%.

Table 8. Number of Hospitals Involved in a Merger or Consolidation by Presence or Absence of a State Hospital Rate Setting Program, 1980–1985

Hospital in/not in a Rate State	Hospitals That Merged		Hospitals That Consolidated		All Hospitals in the United States
	Acquired Hospitals	Acquiring Hospitals	Combining Hospitals	New Hospital Entity	
In a rate state[a]	34%(19)	29%(13)	18%(11)	19%(6)	13%(921)
Not in a rate state	66%(36)	71%(32)	82%(51)	81%(26)	87%(5,981)
Total	100%(55)	100%(45)	100%(62)	100%(32)	100%(6,902)

[a]This includes Massachusetts, Maryland, New Jersey, New York, Connecticut, and Washington.

Table 9. Sources of Gross Patient Revenue of Hospitals Involved in a Merger or Consolidation, 1980–1985[a]

Sources of Gross Patient Revenue	Hospitals That Merged		Hospitals That Consolidated		All Hospitals in the United States
	Acquired Hospitals	Acquiring Hospitals	Combining Hospitals	New Hospital Entity	
Medicare	32%($140,645)	36%($420,974)	37%($235,301)	42%($230,193)	38%($53,662,926)
Medicaid	13%(57,128)	10%(119,898)	9%(60,246)	6%(35,963)	11%(15,221,314)
Commercial	15%(66,422)	18%(203,103)	19%(123,295)	14%(78,735)	21%(30,507,282)
Blue Cross/Blue Shield	18%(79,003)	26%(302,927)	17%(106,200)	23%(129,161)	16%(22,454,236)
Self-pay	8%(34,191)	6%(63,897)	7%(42,324)	7%(39,828)	8%(11,553,592)
Other	14%(63,255)	4%(51,259)	11%(68,502)	8%(44,571)	6%(8,121,518)
Total	100%($440,644)	100%($1,162,058)	100%($635,868)	100%($558,451)	100%($141,520,868)

[a]All numbers in thousands.

D. Financial Characteristics

To examine the short-term overall financial conditions of hospitals that merged or consolidated, a financial ratio analysis of the hospitals' liquidity and profitability was conducted.

Liquidity ratios are used in financial ratio analysis to give an assessment of the hospital's ability to meet its current (i.e., due to reach maturity within one year) financial obligations. Profitability ratios, on the other hand, are used to measure any profit or surplus potential generated within the hospital. Two such profit sources, for example, are patient revenues and the hospital's own investments, which are considered nonoperating sources of revenues.

The most commonly used measure of overall liquidity is the current ratio. This ratio compares all of the hospital's current assets with all current liabilities.

The most commonly used measure of overall profitability is the total margin ratio. This ratio compares the profitability of the hospital by dividing its net income by total revenues. Net income includes profits from both operating and nonoperating sources.

Another commonly used measure of overall profitability is the net-to-gross-patient-revenue ratio. This ratio is calculated by dividing total net patient revenues by total gross patient revenues. This measures the overall potential revenues that are ultimately collected. A hospital's having to write off a large percentage of its revenues may indicate either that insufficient attention is given to bill collection or that the client group may be too poor to pay. Either raises concern about the hospital's long-term financial viability.

These three ratios were chosen for this study because of their widespread use and because data used in their calculation were consistently collected by AHA. The Annual Survey of Hospitals for the years 1975–1984 was the source of data for these ratios.

To compare the financial conditions of hospitals before they combined to their conditions after their merger or consolidation, these ratios were computed for each hospital for the five years preceding and up to four years following their merger or consolidation. These ratios were then standardized (z-scores were calculated using all hospitals in the country as the basis for the scores) to control for changes in the hospital industry during the study years. Also, medians rather than the means were used because of missing data and because outliers in the data set made the means difficult to interpret, especially when the number of cases available was small.

Overall, these analyses indicated that (1) hospitals involved in either mergers or consolidations were financially close to the industry averages in that their median standard scores were usually close to zero; and (2) the general financial effects of mergers or consolidations were small. Given the lack of significant differences, the financial analyses tables are not included in this paper.

In sum, no clear financial gains or losses characterized merging or consolidating hospitals either before or after merger or consolidation. Whatever financial considerations may have played a part in the decisions to merge or consolidate, the actual mergers and consolidations appear not to have had any significant financial effects, at least in the short period covered by this study.

IV. SUMMARY OF RESULTS AND CONCLUSIONS

The purpose of this empirical study has been to contribute in two ways to knowledge regarding recent hospital mergers and consolidations: first, by describing the institutional, locational, and environmental characteristics of hospitals that combined in the six-year period 1980–1985; and, second, by examining whether these combinations, in the short term, resulted in significant overall financial changes in the hospitals.

Several insights emerge from the empirical findings of this study.

First, in terms of institutional characteristics, acquiring and consolidating hospitals were more likely to be community hospitals, while acquired hospitals were more likely to be specialty hospitals, compared to all U.S. hospitals. Most mergers consisted of a large hospital acquiring a small bedsize hospital. For consolidations, a similar pattern occurred, with a large hospital combining with a small hospital. Acquiring and consolidating hospitals were predominately not-for-profit, while relatively more governmental and investor-owned hospitals were acquired. Acquiring hospitals had high occupancy rates, while acquired hospitals had rates like all hospitals in the United States. Consolidations appeared to lead to higher occupancy rates.

Second, in terms of locational characteristics, mergers were disproportionately found in the Middle Atlantic Census Division and metropolitan areas. Consolidations were spread more uniformly throughout the country.

Third, in terms of environmental characteristics, a relatively high proportion of mergers and consolidations took place in rate-setting states. New hospital entities had a relatively large percentage of revenues from Medicare. Acquired hospitals had a relatively large percentage of their revenues from Medicaid. Merging and consolidating hospitals had lower percentages of commercial insurance revenues than all hospitals. In contrast, merging and consolidating hospitals had higher percentages of Blue Cross/Blue Shield revenues than all U.S. hospitals.

Fourth, in terms of financial characteristics, the financial conditions of merged and consolidated hospitals, as measured by their current ratio, total margin ratio, and net-to-gross-patient-revenue ratio, were found to be very similar. In general, hospitals that combined tended to merge or consolidate with hospitals with similar financial ratios. And most hospitals that combined were neither in serious financial trouble nor well off before they merged or consolidated. After the hospitals merged or consolidated, no major financial gains or losses (using the three ratios of the study) were found to occur in the short period of time under investigation.

The findings from this study are limited by the fact that only a short period of time could be examined and by the fact that only three financial ratios were used to examine possible overall financial changes. Further research, focusing on a longer period of time, using these and other financial ratios to examine changes and using more sophisticated multivariate analysis techniques to carefully control for differences, is necessary to more definitively answer the questions of which hospitals merge or consolidate and what financial benefits, if any, are obtained.

ACKNOWLEDGMENTS

David McNeil and Steven Andes were instrumental in developing the computer programs for these analyses as well as in helping to formulate the research approach.

REFERENCES

Finkler, Steven A. and Sandra L. Horowitz (1985), "Merger and Consolidation: An Overview of Activity in Healthcare Organizations." *Healthcare Financial Management* 39(1):19–28.

Starkweather, David B. (1981), *Hospital Mergers in the Making*. Ann Arbor, MI: Health Administration Press.

Treat, Thomas Frank (1973), *A Study of the Characteristics and Performance of Merging Hospitals in the United States*. Ph.D. dissertation, University of Michigan.

HOSPITAL PARTICIPATION IN MULTIHOSPITAL SYSTEMS

Michael A. Morrisey and Jeffrey A. Alexander

I. INTRODUCTION

An increasingly important development in the organization and delivery of health care is the multihospital system (MHS). These organizations, defined as two or more hospitals that are owned, leased, sponsored, or managed by a single corporate entity, encompassed 32% of the nation's hospitals and 36% of all community hospital beds in 1982 [American Hospital Association (AHA), 1983]. It has been suggested that by 1990 the hospital industry will be largely composed of several hundred systems rather than several thousand individual institutions, as is currently the case.

Despite this growth and the subsequent organizational changes it has made in the delivery of health care, relatively little empirical research has been directed to the study of systems. Most of the literature is devoted to nonempirical descriptions of particular systems or to declarations of the potential benefits of systems through economies of scale, access to capital, greater operating efficiency, better response to regulation, and increased ability to attract high-quality administrative and clinical staffs.

Advances in Health Economics and Health Services Research, Vol. 7, pgs. 59–81.
Copyright © 1987 by JAI Press Inc.
All rights of reproduction in any form reserved.
ISBN: 0-89232-573-9

The empirical literature that does exist finds little difference between system and nonsystem hospitals. As Ermann and Gabel (1984) report, while there is some evidence of higher costs in system hospitals, there is no evidence of differential care for the disadvantaged or differences in case mix, and generally no evidence of differences in quality. In fact, the only clear "system declaration" to be suggested by the limited number of studies available is greater access to capital.

The conclusions of the literature, however, must be received with suspicion, as they rest upon at least two critical assumptions:

First, it is implicitly assumed that system participation is the result of some random selection process entered into by hospitals and/or established systems. Hospitals do not randomly enter into MHSs but opt for these arrangements due to a variety of management and market conditions. To the extent that such predisposing conditions and selection factors are not adequately considered, the comparisons between system and freestanding hospitals will be biased. In matched sample studies the bias will be toward no difference.

Second, the literature has given little consideration to the potentially important differences among systems and system hospitals. Systems differ in their ownership, organization, and control of constituent members. For example, systems may own, lease, or contract-manage hospitals, provide close policy direction, or allow considerable institutional autonomy. If factors such as these are significant, then failure to make the appropriate distinction among "system hospitals" will again bias the estimated differences between system and independent hospitals.

The purpose of this study is to explicitly examine the phenomenon of hospitals joining systems. Particularly, we will examine the market and management factors associated with hospital entry in an MHS. We make a distinction between hospitals acquired by systems and hospitals which enter into management contracts and analyze the differences in the factors underlying the entry decisions.

The findings of this investigation have potentially important implications for further research in the area as well as for the likely development of the industry. If entry into systems is a nonrandom event, this implies that systems may have significant effects on hospital performance, costs, and outcomes which have yet to be identified. More fundamentally, it implies that the growth of systems may be limited if the market and management conditions for acquisition or contract management are limited.

The implementation of Medicare prospective payment and the apparent increased price consciousness in health care may fundamentally change the health care environment. If our contentions about the role of market forces are correct, these innovations should lead to changes in the organization of the industry. We begin the ongoing evaluation of these changes by examining whether state rate-setting programs and hospital and physician competition affected the development of systems in the preprospective pricing period.

Next, the existing literature is reviewed in Section II. Section III presents the underlying theoretical issues. This is followed by a discussion of the data and methodology in Section IV. Section V contains the results of the empirical analysis. Section VI contains the conclusions and implications of the investigation.

II.   BACKGROUND

The large and growing literature on multihospital systems has largely ignored issues related to hospital entry into systems. Much of this work, however, is strongly influenced by unstated assumptions regarding such entry patterns.

A.   Assumptions of the Literature

A considerable portion of MHS literature is devoted to describing, advocating, and in a few cases empirically testing the suggested benefits of hospital participation in systems. Writers on the subject have identified at least four general advantages possessed by MHS hospitals as compared to independent hospitals (Lewin and Associates, 1981; Zuckerman, 1979; Mason, 1979;, Cooney and Alexander, 1975; DeVries, 1978): (1) *economic benefits* such as economics of scale and access to capital; (2) *improved personnel and management benefits* such as ability to recruit, train, and retain high-quality medical and administrative staffs, expand patient referral networks, and provide access to administrative specialists to assist in coping with increasingly complex environments; (3) *organizational benefits* due to expansion of the service area, increased market penetration, and organizational survival through reduced financial deficits, manpower shortages, and facilities problems; and (4) *community benefits* such as improved access and quality of care through enhanced resources, lower costs, and improved regional planning.

There have been 18 research studies conducted comparing MHS hospitals and freestanding hospitals on hospital-specific economic performance outcomes (Ermann and Gabel, 1984). Research in this area has demonstrated that systems had somewhat lower staffing ratios, suggesting that there was more efficient use of personnel and that system hospitals experience increased cost of care, particularly under investor-owned operation. Differences on other outcomes are either nonexistent or contradictory (see, for example, Cooney and Alexander, 1975; Lewin and Associates, 1976; Sloan and Vracui, 1983; Patterson and Katz, 1983; Biggs et al., 1980).

Data-based research on personnel and management benefits, organizational benefits, and community benefits of systems are few, and thus no conclusions may be drawn regarding MHS effectiveness in these areas.

The rather unspectacular results of MHS performance research to date could be attributable in part to false assumptions related to patterns of hospital entry into systems. These assumptions are enumerated below.

Hospitals randomly select into systems.   This assumption is virtually universal in MHS research and has the effect of discounting systematic selection factors as a major influence in hospital performance under MHS management. Matching or control variable strategies in MHS research effectively wash out the organizational characteristics associated with entry in an MHS. These assumed that control or matching variables (e.g., length of stay, size, hospital beds per capita) may exercise considerable influence in MHS research if they are associated with commonly used performance measures.

Benefits of system participation are universal and implicitly equated with entry patterns.   Much of the performance-based research on MHS assumes that suggested outcomes of MHS participation are universally sought by hospitals and systems and that entry patterns reflect conditions that motivate hospitals and/or systems to improve performance in theses areas (e.g., poor operating efficiency and inability to recruit qualified personnel).

In fact, the suggested benefits of MHS membership may have little association with conditions that dispose hospitals to join or be selected by systems. For example, hospitals interested in increasing their market share may be less motivated to achieve economics of scale or enhance personnel recruitment. Similarly, as Ermann and Gabel (1984) note, systems may choose to operate only in areas that offer maximum potential for financial success (e.g., low-Medicaid or indigent populations). This suggests that performance research on MHSs must carefully identify and incorporate conditions of entry into systems as part of the performance appraisal. Such conditions influence what performance areas are appropriate for investigation and what hospitals are appropriate for comparison purposes.

All hospitals participate in systems for the same reasons or under the same conditions.   Although this "organizations are all alike" approach is frequently assumed in MHS research, it is dysfunctional to the extent that findings often reflect the situation of the composite hospital, an entity without counterpart in the hospital industry. Further, these general tendencies may wash out the effects of variation in hospital entry patterns on hospital performance.

All systems acquire hospitals for the same reasons and under the same conditions. Systems may employ, as part of their corporate strategy, acquisition criteria that direct them to market themselves in particular geographic areas and/or with hospitals possessing specific, predefined characteristics. To the extent that such corporate strategies influence hospital entry, research on MHS must address and identify those strategies as integral elements of performance appraisal of hospitals on MHS.

B. Literature on Hospital Entry into Multihospital Systems

It is difficult to draw definitive conclusions about MHS entry from the limited body of research in that area. Enough suggestive evidence exists, however, to seriously question the implicit assumptions made in much of the existing MHS performance literature.

Alexander et al. (1985a) used analysis of variance and clustering analysis to develop a taxonomy based on systematic differences in hospitals belonging to secular, nonprofit MHSs. The 366 hospitals in the analysis clustered into 10 distinct groupings based on a set of 12 organizational variables. Groups of hospitals in the owned and leased affiliation categories were more distinct than those in the contract-managed category. These findings suggest that clearly defined and different patterns of entry may occur for hospitals that are bought or leased by systems. External validation of the clustering solution using hospital operating and governance characteristics indicated that owned hospitals are more profitable and more efficient than the leased and contract-managed hospitals. Contract-managed hospitals tended to be smaller and to have boards that were less occupationally representative and less accountable to higher authority.

Geographic and regional patterns of entry are also suggested by Mullner et al. (1981). They found a heavy concentration of system hospital beds in the West and Southwestern states, a lesser concentration in the Middle North Central region, and very low concentration in the New England and Middle Atlantic areas. However, when they disaggregated this distribution according to type of ownership of the MHS beds, different patterns became apparent. Hospital beds in nonprofit systems were distributed broadly; investor-owned systems were concentrated in the West, South, and Southwest. While Mullner offers no explanation for these distributions, the geographic patterns offer evidence that hospital entry into systems is, at least for investor-owned systems, systematic and nonrandom.

From the perspective of the hospital, Townsend (1983) provides case study support for the notion that the circumstances relating to hospital entry into an MHS may vary considerably. Four entrants into investor-owned systems were examined. The two midsize county hospitals studied cited obsolescence of physical plant and capital equipment, coupled with the inability to generate new capital through bond revenues. By contrast, a small nonprofit hospital located in a metropolitan area was financially healthy, but its owners were pessimistic about the future of small institutions in a highly competitive environment. The final hospital in the study, a small osteopathic hospital, was a privately owned institution located in an area deemed to have an excess number of hospital beds.

Corporate acquisition strategies affecting hospital entry into an MHS also have received limited treatment in the literature. Anecdotal data, however, strongly suggest that MHSs, particularly in the investor-owned sector, closely scrutinize potential acquisitions on a number of criteria. Recent articles (Alexander et al., 1985b; Johnson, 1982; Johnson and DiPaolo, 1981) suggest the following:

- Investor-owned systems are more likely to buy hospitals with aged physical plants and then build replacement facilities.
- All systems examine criteria such as growth potential, age of medical staff, and mix of cost- and charge-based patient loads.
- Buyers avoid hospitals with underpriced services because of potential community resentment of substantial markups.
- Buyers attempt to acquire hospitals with low debt-to-equity ratios so that hospital assets may be used as collateral for loans to buy the institution or finance capital improvements or renovations.

Other empirical research provides indirect support to the argument that operational differences between investor-owned and nonprofit systems may influence a system's acquisition strategy and a hospital's decision to join a particular system. Alexander and Fennell (1986), in an analysis of 160 MHSs, found that systems vary in their operating policies, particularly regarding the locus of decision making between headquarters and system hospitals. Decisions related to resource allocation, strategic planning, operations, and administrative accountability were most centralized in nonprofit systems, in geographically concentrated systems, and in systems engaged only in the business of running hospitals.

The literature concerning the effects of payment systems on multihospital system performance and growth is virtually nonexistent. A review of the Mullner et al. (1981) study reveals that investor-owned systems have avoided states with mandatory rate-setting programs. The voluntary chains, however, are represented in these areas. The number of elderly in Florida and the heavy concentration of investor-owned systems in the state suggest that Medicare payment for hospital services may have been an important factor in the growth of systems. These observations suggest that eventual reductions of Medicare payment through prospective payment could retard or redirect at least investor-owned system growth.

On the other hand, Cook, et al. (1983) argued that systems may be more managerially effective in such regulated environments because of economics of scale in administratively dealing with these environmental factors. If so, systems may have a comparative advantage vis-à-vis freestanding hospitals in surviving under such a payment system.

The literature also suggests key differences in entry patterns between hospitals that are acquired or bought by systems, on the one hand, and those that are contract-managed by systems, on the other.

A detailed analysis of the financial characteristics of contract-managed hospitals (Alexander and Lewis, 1985) indicated systematic differences in the financial positions of a group of 90 hospitals prior to entry into contract management arrangements. Relative to traditionally managed hospitals, this "pre-contract-managed" group displayed higher debt ratios, lower current ratios, and lower operating margins. This group of hospitals was comparable to the comparison group on asset turnover, return on assets, and markup. Additional differences in financial ratios were noted when hospitals managed by investor-owned firms, as distinct from nonprofit firms, were compared to the group of traditionally managed hospitals.

A descriptive analysis of hospitals under contract management (Alexander and Lewis, 1984) suggested differences between these hospitals and the population of non-contract-managed, non-MHS hospitals. Contract-managed institutions tended to be smaller, located in rural areas, and disproportionately represented in the West North Central, Mountain, and South Atlantic census regions. This analysis also indicated possible entry patterns based on type of management organization. Investor-owned management organizations, relative to nonprofit organizations, were more likely to manage larger hospitals and urban hospitals. Further, hospitals managed by investor-owned firms tended to dominate in the West South Central and Middle Atlantic regions, while nonprofit management had a much larger market share in the West North Central region.

Finally, the previously discussed study by Alexander et al. (1985a) noted that organizational characteristics of owned and leased MHS hospitals were more clearly defined than contract-managed MHS hospitals. These findings suggest that entry patterns for contract-managed hospitals are distinct from those of acquired hospitals.

III.   THEORETICAL UNDERPINNINGS

We begin the theoretical discussion with an analysis of the decision of a system to acquire a hospital. We then expand the discussion to examine the management contract. We also begin with an assumption of profit-maximizing hospitals and systems. This assumption is later relaxed to allow a more complete discussion of the rationale for contract management.

A. Profit-Maximizing Firms

The acquisition decision of the profit-maximizing system is essentially a comparison of the proposed sales price of the hospital with the expected net present value of its income stream. If the sales price is below the system's estimate of the hospital's net present value, the system acquires the hospital. Net present value (NPV), as calculated in Eq. (1), is simply the sum of expected revenue (R) in each time period (i) less the expected costs in each period (Ci) over the expected life of the hospital (T). Because each time period is farther removed from the sales date (i = 0), the value of the revenue and costs in each period is discounted by the opportunity cost of funds $(1 + r)^i$, where r is the interest rate:

$$NPV = \sum_{i=1}^{T} \frac{R_i - C_i}{(1 + r)^i} . \tag{1}$$

A system will acquire a hospital only if it believes that the stream of net revenue exceeds the asking price of the hospital. The hospital will sell only if the system's bid exceeds its own calculations of net present value. Differences in bid and asking prices arise because of differences in R, C, or r. The system and the hospital may have differing views as to the growth of the market for hospital services, thereby affecting expected revenues and perhaps cost. The system may expect to have lower costs of operating the hospital and thus may expect to receive a larger net revenue flow than does the current owner. (Indeed, this is the presumed raison d'être of the system.) Finally, the system may have a lower cost of capital than does the hospital, perhaps because of lower risk of bankruptcy.[1]

The system's calculation is actually more complex than that of the hospital because the system must consider the indirect effects upon its other member hospitals. It may acquire a teaching hospital, for example, predominately because the perceived high quality and access to the full spectrum of services will increase the profits of all the system's hospitals (Alexander et al., 1985b). In the subsequent discussion, we focus on the acquisition of community hospitals, where the indirect effects are likely to be small.

The net present value formula identifies the idealized information players on both sides of the acquisition will seek to acquire. However, that decision rule is driven by the estimates and expectations of the participants. Those estimates of revenues and costs are based upon the future strength of the hospital's market and the relative abilities of the hospital's and the system's management. Figure 1 heuristically summarizes these market and management forces and their hypothesized effects on acquisition. Market factors are those elements beyond the control of the hospital. They include

Figure 1. The acquisition decision.

MARKET FACTORS

		Favorable	Unfavorable
M A N A G E M E N T	F A C T O R S		
	Strong	???	freestanding
		II	I
		III	IV
	Weak	acquired	???

the composition of the population in the community and its growth, payment systems used by government and private insurers, regulation, and the prices of labor and other inputs. Management factors are all those elements of operation over which the board and its administrative and clinical agents have control. These may include staffing, pricing, collectibles, services offered, marketing, and strategic planning.

If a hospital is in an unfavorable market and run by skilled, highly competent management, as in the upper right quadrant of Figure 1, it is unlikely that a potential buyer can do anything to improve the performance of the hospital. Therefore, a hospital in this quadrant is not a good candidate for acquisition by a system. Alternatively, in the lower left quadrant, because there are typically a wide variety of things the new owner can do to increase the profitability of the hospital, a poorly run hospital in a desirable market is likely to be acquired. In the remaining quadrants the acquisition decision depends upon the relative divergence in expectations between the system and the hospital.

In this profit-maximizing model, contract management will appear only because of a divergence in expectations about the future desirability of the market; particularly, the hospital's view must be more optimistic than that of the system. If expectations of the market are identical, the system will simply use its lower expected operating costs to offer a price acceptable to the hospital. On the other hand, if the hospital has sufficiently higher market expectations, it will reject the buyout option. It will, however, be able to acquire the management expertise through contract. The hospital will pay the price for the management contract and keep the remaining flow of net revenue for itself. This scenario also provides little incentive to enter the management contract for purposes of eventual acquisition by the system (Morrisey and Alexander, 1986).

B. Nonprofit Enterprise

The hospital industry is made up of systems and hospitals that are legally not-for-profit. These firms are generally modeled as maximizing a utility function (Newhouse, 1970; Feldstein, 1971; Sloan, 1981); more colloquially, these hospitals have different missions. Yet, like profit-maximizing organizations, without carefully managing their resources and generating internal surpluses, they are unable to devote resources to their missions (see Long, 1976; Long and Silvers, 1976; and Conrad, 1984).

As a consequence, a nonprofit system will consider the same market and management factors considered by investor-owned firms. Indeed, this is confirmed by our case studies (Alexander et al., 1985b). The weights they attach to particular factors will differ. A Catholic system, for example, may give more weight to the number of Catholics in the community. The upshot of this difference in missions is that nonprofit systems, in selected instances, will be more likely to acquire hospitals in quadrants II and IV than are strictly profit-maximizing firms.

A second implication, developed in more detail elsewhere (Morrisey and Alexander, 1986), is that conflicts in the missions of the system and the hospital provide a strong rationale for the development of management contracts. In this context the contract serves as a mechanism to provide expertise in management without relinquishing the policymaking authority of the hospital's board. As a consequence, we expect to see management contracts disproportionately entered into by systems and hospitals with different missions.

Finally, in the context of the decision to enter a management contract, the mission conflict argument implies that market conditions are only indirectly associated with the decision. The contract decision is based fundamentally upon the skill (or lack of it) on the part of the current management. Market factors matter only in establishing the objectives of the new management and in ensuring that there will be sufficient revenues to cover the management fee.

C. Testable Implications

This model of acquisitions and management contracts leads to a number of testable implications. Because we are limited to data on acquisitions and management contracts occurring in 1982 and 1983, we focus on three:

1. Systems will acquire poorly managed hospitals located in favorable markets.

2. Hospitals are more likely to be acquired by systems with similar missions.
3. Management contracts will tend to exist in poorly managed hospitals; market factors are largely irrelevant.

IV. METHODS AND DATA

A. Methods

The theory offers a very straightforward empirical model to be estimated. It is summarized in Eq. (2):

$$MHS = f(MKT^x, MGT^x, Mission), \qquad (2)$$

that is, the decision to affiliate with a multihospital system is a function of the market conditions expected to prevail over the life of the affiliation (MKT^x), the expected course of management factors which would prevail if the hospital continued its present course (MGT^x), and the respective missions of the system and hospital.

We examine two variants of system affiliation. In the first, the system acquires the hospital. Here we hypothesize that the probability of entering into a system increases with the expected improvement in market conditions but decreases with the competence of the existing management. In the second instance the hospital enters into a management contract with the system. In this case we anticipate that the probability of the formation of a management contract will decrease with the competence of the existing management. We hypothesize no clear relationship between expected market factors and formation of a management contract.

Because the dependent variables are dichotomous, ordinary least squares estimates, while unbiased, are not of minimum variance. Further, because of the characteristics of our sample design, both ordinary least squares and a probit specification will lead to biased coefficient estimates. A logit model, therefore, was employed to minimize the effect of the bias.

Ermann and Gabel (1984) observe that there are relatively few acquisitions or management contracts formed in any one year; generally on the order of 150 hospitals are involved. To examine these vis-à-vis some 3300 freestanding hospitals in each year creates problems of estimation efficiency and cost. To overcome these problems we employed a choice-based sampling strategy. In essence it involves drawing all hospitals which joined a system in the relevant year plus a random sample of nonjoiners. As Maddala (1983) and Amemiya (1985) make clear, the use of logit analysis in this situation results in increased precision in the estimates and bias limited to the intercept term.

Because expectations in Eq. (2) are unobservable, we adopt the common assumption that they are an unbiased function of past trends. Thus, we measure market and management factors as the change in the relevant variables over the five years preceding the acquisition or management contract. Finally, we must acknowledge a misspecification of the mission variables. While we include proxies for the hospital's mission, the data set is not large enough to allow separate estimates for each type of system.

B. Data

Data for this investigation were obtained from three principle sources: (1) the 1978, 1979, 1982, and 1983 AHA Annual Surveys of Hospitals; (2) the 1983 Area Resource File; and (3) the 1983 AHA Multihospital System Validation File. The Annual Surveys are recognized as a basic source of data on U.S. hospitals and provide information for all U.S. hospitals on (1) facilities and services provided by the hospital; (2) hospital ownership management and control; (3) the financial position of the hospital—revenue, expenses, assets, and liabilities; (4) hospital personnel; and (5) inpatient beds and utilization. Items on the Annual Survey are modified slightly from year to year, but those relevant to this investigation are consistent across years, permitting analysis of change.

The Area Resource File (ARF) is a compendium of data sources that encompasses a wide range of health and population characteristics. Sources for these data include the AHA, American Medical Association (AMA), American Dental Association (ADA), American Nurses Association (ANA), U.S. Bureau of the Census, National Center for Health Statistics, and Social Security Administration, among others. Data are specified for the 3077 U.S. counties and are compatible for cross-county comparisons. Most data items are available for multiple years, allowing for assessments of change in health and population variables over time. General content areas of the ARF include county demographic characteristics, family characteristics, health occupations, hospitals and other health facilities, health professionals, and socioeconomic factors.

The MHS validation file is a comprehensive listing of all multihospital systems and their member hospitals (approximately 1850) as of 1983. The file contains information on ownership of the system, the location of its headquarters, affiliation of each of the member hospitals with the system (e.g., owned, contract-managed, or sponsored), and the year hospital became affiliated with the system. The AHA defines a MHS as two or more hospitals that are owned, leased, contract-managed, or sponsored by a separate administrative entity. It is a simple matter to decompose this definition into its constituent forms of affiliation.

Table 1.   Hospital Entering Systems by Year and Type of Affiliation

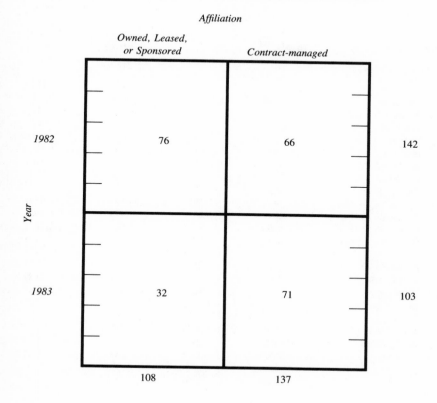

Affiliation

	Owned, Leased, or Sponsored	Contract-managed	
1982	76	66	142
1983	32	71	103
	108	137	

Year

C.   Sample

The sample for this investigation consisted of all 245 short-term community hospitals that were acquired by or entered into a management contract with a multihospital system in 1982 or 1983. Table 1 presents the distribution of these hospitals by year and affiliation status.

As a comparison group, a randomly selected group of 735 freestanding, short-term community hospitals were added to the data set. These hospitals represent three times the number of hospitals entering systems during the study period. They were drawn from the universe of never-system hospitals in the years corresponding to system entry (i.e., 426 in 1982 and 309 in 1983). For missing values we interpolated on the basis on the basis of pre- and postreported data prior to calculating the five-year change. We deleted observations for which interpolation was not possible. This resulted in an

Table 2.   Means and Standard Deviations

	Acquisition		Contract Management	
	Mean	Std. Dev.	Mean	Std. Dev.
Acquistion	.264		—	
Management Contract	—		.242	
Medicare	.412	(.102)	.415	(.112)
Medicaid	.084	(.061)	.084	(.071)
Private Insurance	.373	(.112)	.372	(.112)
Δ Surgeon/Pop.	.037	(.072)	.039	(.068)
Δ FP/Pop.	.022	(.098)	.013	(.088)
Δ Beds/Pop.	− .004	(1.674)	− .143	(1.565)
Δ No. Hospitals	− .577	(2.678)	− .415	(2.410)
Δ HMO/Pop.	.011	(.051)	.009	(.039)
Δ Unemp. Rate	3.806	(3.326)	3.857	(3.158)
Δ Income/Pop. (100s)	35.901	(11.251)	34.946	(10.810)
Δ Population (100,000s)	.289	(1.254)	.174	(1.109)
Δ Percent Aged ≥ 65	9.570	(11.315)	9.823	(11.187)
Rate-Setting Years	.814	(2.500)	1.163	(2.999)
Con Years	10.510	(18.821)	10.320	(19.263)
Existing Sys.	.765	(.418)	.739	(.431)
% Docs 45–54	.434	(.246)	.452	(.264)
Teaching	.012	(.060)	.013	(.061)
Beds (100s)	1.536	(1.627)	1.518	(1.560)
Gov't Hosp.	.339	(.473)	.387	(.487)
Inv. Owned	.094	(.307)	.039	(.216)
Fac. & Serv.	13.564	(8.091)	13.578	(7.795)
Δ Rev/Exp[a]	.000	(.119)	.000	(.151)
Δ Payroll/Exp[a]	.000	(.056)	.000	(.055)
Δ Occ. Rate[a]	.000	(.125)	.000	(.121)
N	392		491	

[a] Residual of subsidiary equation.
Δ Five-year change.

acquisition file of 392 hospitals and a contract management file of 491 observations.

D.   Empirical Model

The variables used in the analysis are summarized in Table 2. The particular variables are derived from discussions with system executives (Alexander et al., 1985b), the available literature, and concerns of data availability. Our measures of market factors are defined at the county level and usually measured as the five-year change.

The measures include hospital insurance coverage measured as the proportions of hospital gross patient revenue from Medicare, Medicaid, and private insurance. These values are measured at the hospital level because hospital catchment areas are believed to be fairly stable and because the data were unavailable prior to 1980. Our assertion is that larger proportions of private insurance coverage (and to a lesser extent greater Medicare coverage) increased both the fees and volumes of service the hospital provides. This increases the anticipated net present value and therefore increases probability of acquisition.

As the number of physicians per capita increases we anticipate an increase in the demand for hospital services. Because surgeons are generally dependent upon hospitals and family practitioners are sometimes thought of as substitutes for hospital service, we include two measures: the changes in the number of surgeons and family practitioners per 1000 population.

Other things equal, a growing hospital capacity in the market will decrease the returns to hospital care and the desirability of acquiring a hospital. We measure changes in hospital capacity as the change in the number of nonfederal hospital beds per 1000 population and the change in the number of hospitals.

We also include a measure of the change in health maintenance organization (HMO) market share on the assumption that such growth may be a proxy for competitive changes that may be occurring in the health care market.

Growth in the population, its income, and its age increase the demand for hospital care and should increase the expected net present value of the hospital and its probability of acquisition. We measure these as the change in the population, per capita income, the unemployment rate, and the proportion of the population aged 65 and over.

As we noted in the background section (Section II), there is speculation, and some theory, that the extent of regulation will influence the acquisition strategies of systems. We examine two programs. State-run rate-setting programs and certificate-of-need legislation are measured as the number of years each was in effect as of the year of acquisition.

We also attempt to capture some element of the political climate toward systems in the state. Two measures were used. First, a binary variable taking the value "one" if there was an investor-owned system hospital in the state at the time of acquisition. If so, it implies that any political fight over investor-owned systems had already been fought in the state. Following Morrisey and Ashby (1982), we also include the proportion of physicians in the state aged 45–54. The argument is that these physicians have established practices and are likely to be politically "well connected." If systems are perceived as disturbing the status quo, these physicians potentially have the most to gain or lose.

Management factors are particularly difficult to measure. We use a series of changes in hospital performance in a recursive system to obtain proxies for these critical measures. Specifically, we include three available measures of performance: the ratio of net revenue to expenditures, the ratio of payroll to expenditures, and the occupancy rate. Each is measured as the five-year change prior to the year of affiliation with a system. The first is taken as an overall measure of hospital performance. Controlling for market factors, growth in the return on operations is indicative of strong management. The second is a measure of ability to cope with labor issues. The expected sign, however, is unclear. A declining ratio may reflect on inability to attract sufficient staff; an increasing ratio may reflect wasteful overstaffing. We assert only that management of labor issues is important to a determination of whether to acquire or contract manage a particular hospital. Third, we include a measure of the change in the occupancy rate of the facility. This measure is intended to capture management's ability to market its services and appropriately staff its bed stock. An increasing occupancy rate, given market conditions, is indicative of stronger management and reduced likelihood of either acquisition or contract management.

Since such performance measures are a function of both market conditions and underlying management factors, their direct inclusion will measure something more than management skill and will also bias our market measures. To overcome this we estimate a series of three subsidiary equations, one for each of our measures. In these equations we regress the change in performance on the previously discussed market variables. We then enter the residuals in our system affiliation equation.

Finally, because issues of mission matter to the acquisition or contract management decision, we include five variables that attempt to identify the goals of the institution. That is, we include measures of ownership, bed size, teaching status (residents per bed), and the number of a selected set of facilities and services offered by the hospital. These were measured in the year of affiliation.

V.   RESULTS

The results are summarized in Table 3. It is immediately evident that acquisition decisions and contract management decisions are fundamentally different. We focus first on the market factors, then on the management and control mission variables.

It is apparent that the mix of insurance coverage in the hospital's catchment area plays an important role in the acquisition decision. As the proportion of private insurance or Medicaid coverage increases there is a statistically significant increase in the odds of acquisition. The results imply that a 1-percentage-point increase in these coverages increases the probability of an acquisition by .9% and .8%, respectively. In contrast, the

Table 3. Regression Results of Hospital Entry into Multihospital Systems

		Acquisition		Management Contract	
		Coef.	Std. Error	Coef.	Std. Error
	Constant	−6.685***	(1.890)	−.068	(1.305)
	Medicare	2.960	(2.004)	−.952	(1.351)
	Medicaid	5.144*	(2.934)	.822	(2.003)
	Private Insurance	4.343**	(1.958)	−.417	(1.448)
Δ	Surgeon/Pop.	−1.416	(2.085)	1.634	(1.779)
Δ	FP/Pop.	−.465	(1.401)	−.673	(1.220)
Δ	Beds/Pop.	−.043	(.091)	−.098	(.089)
Δ	No. Hospitals	.006	(.071)	.190	(.169)
Δ	HMO/Pop.	1.852	(2.385)	1.791	(3.037)
Δ	Unemp.	.055	(.045)	−.001	(.041)
Δ	Income/Pop.	.037***	(.014)	−.015	(.013)
Δ	Population	−.085	(.163)	−.388	(.286)
Δ	Percent Aged ≥ 65	−.013	(.012)	.003	(.010)
	Rate-Setting Years	−.143*	(.083)	.034	(.049)
	Con Years	.001	(.008)	−.020*	(.010)
	Existing Sys.	.536	(.399)	.705**	(.317)
	% Docs 45–54	−.768	(.684)	−.112	(.423)
	Teaching	−4.399	(3.930)	−3.156	(3.733)
	Beds	.082	(.133)	−.203	(.144)
	Gov't Hosp.	.407	(.336)	.419*	(.249)
	Inv. Owned	2.331***	(.467)	−.566	(.687)
	Fac. & Serv.	.016	(.027)	−.028	(.023)
Δ	Rev/Exp[a]	.243	(1.208)	.207	(.738)
Δ	Payroll/Exp[a]	−5.841*	(2.440)	−2.437	(1.980)
Δ	Occ. Rate[a]	.148	(1.057)	.276	(.909)
	R	.236		.071	
	Model Chi-Square	71.95, 24 d.f.		50.72, 24 d.f.	
	Fraction Concordant Pairs	.761		.703	

Δ Five-year change.
[a] Residual of subsidiary equation.
* Significant at 90% confidence level, chi-square test.
** Significant at 95% confidence level, chi-square test.
*** Significant at 99% confidence level, chi-square test.

contract management equation offers no statistically significant insurance effects. The Medicaid result is unexpected. It may reflect the interest of some systems to acquire an intercity "franchise" for the purpose of building a new facility in the suburbs (see Alexander et al., 1985b).

The physician and hospital capacity measures have no statistically significant effects. However, there is some evidence that system acquisitions are attracted to markets with fewer hospitals. In earlier analyses (which relied on 1982/83 "levels" of the independent variables rather than changes) there was a strong negative relationship between increases in the number of hospitals and the probability of acquisition. Here, a more rapid decline in the number of hospitals is associated with slightly increased odds of entry.

More rapid growth in HMOs is associated with increases in acquisitions and management contracts, but the results are without statistical significance at the usual levels. This finding is of interest because it is sometimes suggested that systems would avoid HMO markets and focus on less competitive and (presumably) more profitable markets. We find no evidence of this.

The sociodemographic changes in the community have an impact on acquisitions but not on contract management. Consistent with expectations, a more rapid increase in per capita income is associated with an increase in acquisitions. An increasing rate of unemployment is also positively associated with acquisitions. Since insurance coverage and a number of other income and demographic factors are controlled, the variable may be capturing declining labor costs. Finally, while population growth and aging had positive effects in earlier "levels" equations, their trends have no statistically significant effects on either acquisitions or contract management. It may be that systems were entering large, established markets as opposed to growing markets in the 1982/83 period.

The effects of regulation had significant effects on both acquisitions and management contracts. As we speculated, state-run rate-setting programs appear to be effective mechanisms for inhibiting the growth of system acquisitions. Presumably the reduced payment levels reduce the expected net present value and the probability of acquisition. Interestingly, rate setting was positively associated with contract management, albeit not at the conventional levels of significance. This finding offers some support for the Cook et al. (1983) argument that systems offer some economies of scale in dealing with regulatory apparatus. This view of the results suggests that while reimbursement effects dominate, there may indeed be management economies in dealing with regulation.

The certificate-of-need (CON) results offer some of the first evidence that the programs have affected hospital market behavior. Salkever and Bice (1976) found that the programs did reduce beds, but also increased the amount of capital per bed. Our results suggest that the existing laws may be sheltering existing capacity. That is, an increase in the number of years a CON program was in existence is significantly associated with both more acquisitions and fewer management contracts. Suppose over time that the demand for hospital services has increased but the CON authority has been effective in preventing new capacity from entering the market. This implies that existing providers could be obtaining rents because of the higher prices or the relatively leaner services they are providing. These rents increase the net present value of a hospital and attract acquisitions. At the same time, the increased demand coupled with limits on the entry of new capacity suggests that less adept management can survive as a result of the market growth. Thus, fewer management contracts are written.

Finally, we included two measures of the political environment. The strength of the established physician block had no statistically significant effect, although it was of the expected sign. Similarly, the prior presence of an investor-owned chain hospital in the state had no statistically significantly effect on the odds of acquisition. It is associated, however, with a higher odds of contract management. One explanation is that the investor-owned hospital increased competition or the fear of it. Alternatively the presence may have lead to increased hospital board knowledge of contract management potential.

Using a likelihood ratio test, we are able to reject the null hypothesis that market factors are irrelevant to the acquisition decision at the 90% confidence level. The contract management equation does not allow rejection of the null hypothesis at this level of confidence.

Turning to the management variables, we find only limited success in explaining acquisition or contract management decisions. An increase in the change in the revenue-to-expenditures ratio is positively associated with both acquisitions and management contracts, suggesting that systems are affiliating with improving hospitals. This same finding is obtained with respect to increases in the change in occupancy rate.

The results with respect to the payroll-to-expenditure ratio, however, do suggest that management difficulties enter the affiliation decision. The greater the increase in the labor-to-total-expenditures ratio, the lower are the odds of both acquisition and management contract. This suggests that anticipated low future levels of staffing are regarded as an area of potential improvement by a system. Alternatively, the decrease in the labor ratio may suggest better staffing decisions being made by the hospital. This interpretation would then be consistent with those of profitability and occupancy.

However, taken as a group, the management variables do not allow the rejection of the null hypothesis of no effect. It may be that within good markets, management factors of particular hospitals are irrelevant. Given the effort that systems devote to obtaining hospital-specific data in the acquisition process, at least, it seems more likely that we have poor measures of management.

Finally, the control mission variables suggest a pattern in the types of hospitals which affiliate with systems. We find that in the 1982/83 period, investor-owned hospitals were significantly more likely to be acquired by systems and less likely to enter into management contracts than were government or private voluntary hospitals. This is consistent with our theoretical expectations. Government-run hospitals were most likely to enter into management contracts. In contrast to the more recent anecdotal accounts, teaching hospitals in this period were far less likely to affiliate. There were no statistically significant relationships between hospital size or the facilities and services offered and system affiliation.

VI.   CONCLUSIONS AND IMPLICATIONS

It is dangerous to draw hard and fast conclusions on basis of data from two years. Nonetheless, the analysis yields four principal findings:

First, the factors underlying the acquisition and contract management of hospitals are fundamentally different. Acquisitions, in large measure, are a function of the market in which the hospital operates. Management contracts seem to exist almost independently of the market conditions, although there is some weak evidence that they exist in less desirable markets. Management factors, to the extent we could measure them, are only modestly associated with system affiliation.

Second, within the category of market factors it appears that the extent of private and Medicaid hospital insurance coverage and growth in income are particularly important to the likelihood of acquisition.

Third, regulation of hospital reimbursement and construction seems to have been a significant factor in the dispersion of both acquisitions and management contracts. State rate setting reduces the probability of systems acquiring hospitals in the state but has a small positive influence on the development of management contracts. CON regulation, in contract, increased the likelihood of acquisitions and decreased contract management. We interpret these findings as consistent with rate setting reducing hospital profitability and CON limiting hospital bed capacity, thereby increasing the potential profitability of a hospital in a regulated market.

Fourth, there is weak support for the view that systems acquire hospitals in which management has been improving its ability to cope with its environment.

From this analysis we draw several tentative conclusions. First, systems are unlikely to take over the industry through the acquisition of hospitals. Since systems appear to focus on market fundamentals, it is only those hospitals in favorable economic environments that are "at risk." This also suggests that systems are not and will not become the saviors of public general, rural, or other community hospitals. Such hospitals tend to be in declining markets or to have unfavorable payor mixes. There is some evidence, however, that systems will acquire hospitals with larger Medicaid loads. One interpretation of this finding is that these acquisitions are made with the intent to rebuild the facility in a more favorable neighborhood. Alternatively, the finding may reflect the willingness of non-profit-maximizing systems to acquire hospitals for nonmarket reasons. The finding may also reflect some unidentified third factor. Systems may acquire urban hospitals, for example, which coincidentally have higher Medicaid loads.

Our findings suggest, too, that contract management is not, in general, a stepping stone to acquisition. As we argue elsewhere, in the 1976–1983 period only 24 management contracts were converted to system ownership (Morrisey and Alexander, 1986). The reasons for this observation are apparent from this study; unless the managed hospital is in a favorable market, there is little motivation for the acquisition.

Further, our regulation results raise interesting questions of the patterns of industry development as CON programs and rate-setting programs are phased out but the Medicare prospective payment system (PPS) and more price-competitive health delivery systems emerge. The scaling back of rate-setting programs suggests that hospital chains may enter the Northeast, and the elimination of CON provisions implies that hospital markets will become more risky. The PPS and competitive elements offer lower payment, more risk, but potentially more profit for efficient providers. Since our results suggest that the acquisition drive has been fueled by the ability to identify favorable markets and not the potential to improve operations, it seems likely that the hospital acquisition process will slow as a result of the changes in payment strategy.

The finding that the acquisition decision is apparently being driven by underlying market factors calls into question much of the comparative literature on system performance. Since entry is not random, the characteristics underlying the entry decision should be accounted for in analyses of system and nonsystem performance.

This study is among the first to examine the patterns of entry in multihospital systems and has been limited to entrants in the 1982/83 period. As such, more than the usual call for further research is warranted. It is important to know whether the entry patterns observed here are similar to those in earlier and latter periods. Further, our theory suggests that profit-maximizing and utility-maximizing firms should enter somewhat different markets and have systematically different contract managed clients. A larger data set spanning more years is necessary to test these hypotheses.

Our results do suggest, however, the comparative studies of system performance should be reconsidered. To no one's surprise, systems do not randomly select hospitals with which to affiliate. As such, matched sample studies may be missing significant differences in the performance of system and nonsystem hospitals.

Finally, our study highlights the need for more research into the development of empirical measures of management. For research purposes—not to mention business reasons—such measures would aid the understanding and operation of firms.

ACKNOWLEDGMENTS

This study was funded by Grant No. HS05264 from the National Center for Health Services Research and Health Care Technology Assessment. The computer work was completed while we were with the Hospital Research and Educational Trust; we thank them for their continued interest. The opinions and conclusions expressed herein are solely our own, however. Bonnie Lewis and Richard Hahn provided excellent research assistance.

NOTE

1. In a world of reasonably available information and unbiased evaluation by the hospital and the system one would expect the pattern of acquisitions to be random, reflecting only errors of expectation. It is the differences in costs of operation and "indirect benefits" to the systems overall performance that lead to systematic patterns of acquisition.

REFERENCES

Alexander, Jeffrey, James Anderson, and Bonnie Lewis (1985a), "Toward Empirical Classification of Hospitals in Multihospital Systems." *Medical Care* 23(7):913–932.
Alexander, Jeffrey and Mary Fennell (1986), "Patterns of Decisionmaking in Multihospital Systems." *Journal of Health and Social Behavior* 27(1).
Alexander, Jeffrey and Bonnie Lewis (1984), "Hospital Contract Management: A Comparative Analysis." *Health Services Research* 19(4):447–461.
Alexander, Jeffrey and Bonnie Lewis (1985), "Hospital Contract Management: Financial Characteristics of For-Profit and Not-for-Profit Operations." *Inquiry* 21:230–242.
Alexander, Jeffrey, Bonnie Lewis, and Michael A. Morrisey (1985b), "Acquisition Strategies of Multihospital Systems." *Health Affairs* 4(3):49–66.
Amemiya, Takeshi (1985), *Advanced Econometrics*. Cambridge, MA: Harvard University Press.
American Hospital Association (1983), *Directory of Multihospital Systems*. Chicago: AHA.
Biggs, Erol L., John E. Kralewski, and G. Brown (1980), "A Comparison of Contract-Managed and Traditionally-Managed Non-Profit Hospitals." *Medical Care* 18(7):585–596.
Cook, Karin S, Stephen M. Shortell, Douglas A. Conrad, and Michael A. Morrisey (1983), "A Theory of Organizational Response to Regulation: The Case of Hospitals." *Academy of Management Review* 8(2):193–205.
Cooney, James and Thomas Alexander (1975), *Multi-Hospital Systems: An Evaluation*. Chicago: Hospital Research and Educational Trust and Northwestern University.
Conrad, Douglas A. (1984), "Return on Equity to Not-for-Profit Hospitals: Theory and Implications." *Health Service Research* 19(1):41–64.
DeVries, Robert (1978), "Strength in Numbers." *Hospitals, J.A.H.A.* 92(March):81–89.
Ermann, Daniel and Jon Gabel (1984), "Multi-Hospital Systems: Issues and Empirical Findings," *Health Affairs* 3(3):50–64.
Feldstein, Martin S. (1971), "Hospital Cost Inflation: A Study of Nonprofit Price Dynamics." *American Economic Review* 61:853–872.
Johnson, Donald (1982), "Buyers Picky in Growing Market." *Modern Health Care* (May):86–93.

Johnson, Donald and Vincent DiPaalo (1981), "Nonprofits Compete Effectively with Investor-Owned Contract Firms." *Modern Health Care* (April):84–86.

Lewin and Associates (1976), *A Study of Investor-Owned Hospitals.* Chicago: Health Services Foundation.

Lewin, Lawrence, Robert Denson and Rhea Mangolies (1981), "Investor-Owned and Non-Profits Differ in Economic Performance." *Hospitals* 13(55):52–58.

Long, Hugh W. (1976), "Valuation As a Criterion in Not-for-Profit Decision Making." *Health Care Management Review* (Summer):134–152.

Long, Hugh W. and J. B. Silvers (1976), "Health Care Reimbursement Is Federal Taxation of Tax-Exempt Providers." *Health Care Management Review* (Winter):9–23.

Maddala, C. (1983), *Limited-Dependent and Qualitative Variables in Econometrics.* New York: Cambridge University Press.

Mason, Scott (1980), "Greater Access and Lower Costs with Multihospital Systems." *Hospital Financial Management* (May):58–64.

Morrisey, Michael A. and S. Cynthia Ashby (1982), "An Empirical Analysis of HMO Market Share." *Inquiry* 19(2):136–149.

Morrisey, Michael A. and Jeffrey A. Alexander (1986), "Hospital Acquisition or Contract Management: A Theory of Strategic Choice." *Health Care Management Review* (forthcoming).

Mullner, Ross, Calvin Byrne, and Joseph Jubal (1981), "Multihospital Systems in the United States: A Geographical Overview." *Social Science in Medicine* 15:353–359.

Newhouse, Joseph P. (1970), "Toward a Theory of Nonprofit Institutions: An Economic Model of a Hospital." *American Economic Review* 60:64–73.

Patterson, Robert V. and Hallie M. Katz (1983), "Investor-Owned and Not-For-Profit Hospitals." *New England Journal of Medicine* (August 11):58–64.

Salkever, David and Thomas Bice (1976), "The Impact of Certificate-of-Need Controls on Hospital Investment." *Milbank Memorial Fund Quarterly Health and Society* 54(1):185–214.

Sloan, Frank A. (1981), "Regulation and the Rising Cost of Hospital Care." *Review of Economics and Statistics* 63(4):479–487.

Sloan, Frank A. and Robert A. Vraciu (1983), "Investor-Owned and Not-for-Profit Hospitals: Addressing Some Issues." *Health Affairs* 2(1):25–37.

Townsend, Jessica (1983), "When Investor-Owned Corporations Buy Hospitals: Some Issues and Concerns." In B. Gray (ed.), *The New Health Care For Profit: Doctors and Hospitals in a Competitive Environment.* Washington, DC: National Academy Press.

Zuckerman, Howard (1979), *Multi-Institutional Hospital Systems.* Chicago: Hospital Research and Educational Trust.

CAPITAL MARKETS AND THE GROWTH OF MULTIHOSPITAL SYSTEMS

Frank A. Sloan, Michael A. Morrisey, and
Joseph Valvona

I. INTRODUCTION

The American Hospital Association (AHA) defines a system hospital as
one that is owned, leased, sponsored, or contract-managed by an outside
organization (Alexander et al., 1985). One of the dominant trends in the
U.S. hospital industry of the late 1970s and the 1980s is the growth in the
number of hospitals affiliated with a multihospital system. The number of
beds in multihospital systems grew at an annual rate of 3.0% from 1975
to 1982 (Ermann and Gabel, 1984). Investor-owned system beds grew at
a 5.3% rate compared to a 3.5% rate for nonprofit systems. As of 1982,
systems controlled 33% of the community hospitals in the United States.
While some argue that this definition of systems is too broad, these rates
are substantially below the growth projections sometimes forecast for systems, and they nonetheless reflect a steady conversion of independent
hospitals into multihospital system members. Further, the more rapid increase on the part of investor-owned chains suggests that investor-owned
systems may one day dominate the industry. That dominance, however,
would at best be far in the future. The essential question raised by these

Advances in Health Economics and Health Services Research, Vol. 7, pgs. 83–109.
Copyright © 1987 by JAI Press Inc.
All rights of reproduction in any form reserved.
ISBN: 0-89232-573-9

figures is why systems have grown. A related question is why the investor-owned chains have experienced more rapid growth, at least in terms of numbers of beds.

A number of hypotheses have been offered. Economies of scale in production and superior management have often been advanced as rationales (Dorehfest, 1981; Bennett and Ahrendt, 1981; Lewin and Associates, 1981). However, while sufficient to lead to system ownership, these explanations are not necessary conditions. The common practice of entering into management contracts for service sharing are oft-used mechanisms for acquiring these advantages without relinquishing autonomy (Morrisey and Alexander, 1985). A more classic explanation is that the identification of a residual claimant allows the investor-owned system, if not the nonprofit system, to be more efficient. The existing literature, however, generally has not found that investor-owned system hospitals have lower operating costs (Sloan, 1987).

The tentative conclusion reached by Ermann and Gabel (1984) was that systems enjoyed greater access to capital. That is, systems could attract capital at a lower cost. This conclusion, however, was based only upon comparisons of bond ratings. Hernandez and Howie (1979) reported that 78.2% of system tax-exempt debt was rated A+ or better in the 1976/77 period compared to 41.9% for all hospitals. Ermann and Gabel (1984) reported 61% of system tax-exempt debt was so rated in the 1978–1982 period. By comparison, only 18% of independent hospital bonds were A+ or better. Two issues are critical in interpreting these data. First, can independent hospitals secure cheaper nonbond debt, such as bank loans? Does a self-selection underlie the bond ratings data? In this context, selection could mean that organizations with a comparative advantage in securing funds from bonds are rated while others with comparative advantages in other debt (e.g., direct loans) or equity markets do not enter the bond market. Second, do different bond ratings truly reflect differences in the cost of capital?

The issue of investor-owned vs. nonprofit system access to capital is even less well understood. In 1983, an American Hospital Association task force was unable to identify clear net advantages in access to capital by investor-owned and nonprofit hospitals (AHA, 1983, p. 11). Recent interviews of system executives, however, revealed very different perceptions about the relative access to capital by investor-owned and nonprofit systems. Alexander et al. (1985) reported that officials of nonprofit systems believed they paid a higher price for capital. Moreover, unlike investor-owned executives, those running nonprofit chains found capital to be an immediate constraint on further growth.

The purpose of this study then is threefold: (1) to identify the cost of debt capital to the hospital industry; (2) to compare the cost of debt capital across hospital ownership and chain status; and (3) to analyze the differences in the cost of debt, with particular emphasis on measures associated with the risk of the institution.

To understand the role of capital markets in the growth of multihospital systems, we conduct new empirical analysis to address nine specific questions:

1. How do particular types of system hospitals compare with nonsystem hospitals in terms of various measures of short-term and long-term debt and profitability?
2. To what extent have hospitals differed in their sources of debt?
3. Has the cost of debt capital differed between system and independent hospitals?
4. What has been the trend in the relative cost of debt capital?
5. What is the effect of bond ratings on the cost of debt capital?
6. Can hospital characteristics predict hospital bond ratings?
7. Is the cost of debt capital dependent upon the hospital's debt-to-equity ratio, and, if so, how responsive is cost of capital to the degree of hospital leverage?
8. Do hospitals dependent on cost-based reimbursement pay more or less for debt?
9. What effect have mandatory hospital rate-setting programs had on the cost of debt capital to hospitals?

The following section reviews the state of knowledge on hospital cost of capital and considers why cost of debt may differ between system and independent hospitals and between investor-owned and nonprofit organizations. Section III describes the data used in the study. Tabulations based on these data are presented in Section IV. Particular attention is given to the sources of hospital debt, differences in hospital bond ratings, and a financial ratio analysis of hospitals by ownership and chain status. Section V presents results of regression analysis of hospital bond ratings and the yield on hospital debt. Section VI discusses the findings and policy implications.

II. BACKGROUND

Even though the market for capital is national, the cost of debt to various firms in an industry differs for reasons internal and external to the firm. Internal reasons pertain to the probability of defaulting on interest and principal payments as well as lower transactions cost in securing debt capital.

Hospital systems are often said to have both lower risk and lower transactions costs. First, the system has a larger revenue and asset base arising from its several hospitals. Thus, it is less dependent upon a single source of patient demand and presents less of a risk to a lender.[1] Second, the depth of management expertise in the system is seen as an advantage over independent hospitals in dealing with regulatory and competitive pressures. This again lessens risk. Third, the size of the system implies that it will be in the capital market more often. Large size may permit a secondary market in the system's debt to be established, increasing the liquidity of the debt and thereby reducing the risk to a bond holder. Finally, large systems may be more powerful negotiators with third-party payers, private and public, again reducing operating risk.

The size of the system's capital demands may also allow it to reduce the transactions costs of acquiring debt obligations. The system, for example, can pool several projects into a single large bond offering. It can time its entry into the market more easily due to the greater availability of short-term financing, and it can carry more debt without violating the covenants of prior debt obligations.

Externally, the hospital industry has a number of unique characteristics which lead to interhospital differences in the cost of capital, and particularly to differences in the cost of debt.

First, unlike investor-owned hospitals, nonprofit hospitals do not pay a corporate income tax. This tax raises the overall cost of capital to investor-owned hospitals; the tax deductibility feature reduces its cost of debt relative to equity.

Second, virtually all nonprofit hospitals and systems are able to offer tax-exempt bonds, either directly or through a state or local finance authority. This lowers the cost of debt to such hospitals. This difference is mitigated somewhat by the tax-exempt industrial development bonds available to investor-owned hospitals and systems. Historically, restrictive bond covenants and high transactions costs have made this source of capital too expensive (Cohodes and Kinkaid, 1984, pp. 51–53).

Finally, third-party cost-based payment systems subsidize the use of debt. There are several factors to consider. First, cost-based payment reduces the risk of default since the third-party reimburser agrees to pay the cost of care. For this reason, hospitals and systems with greater proportions of cost-based payors should face lower interest rates. Mitigating this subsidy, many cost-based payors do not recognize cost of equity (Long, 1976; Conrad, 1984). Medicare and Medicaid recognize a cost of equity for for-profit but not nonprofit hospitals. As a result, nonprofit organizations are likely to borrow more than for-profit hospitals at the same interest rate as the proportion of revenue from cost-based payer sources increases. The higher debt-to-equity ratio should in turn raise the interest rate. The fact that cost-based payers guarantee payment on "their" share of debt may reduce the incentive that cost-based dependent hospitals have to search for low-cost debt. Finally, to the degree that cost-based reimbursement serves as a cost-containment device, wherein certain costs are disallowed, the programs may increase the cost of debt capital.

Rate-setting programs may be expected to raise the cost of debt; to the extent that they reduce payment levels, they increase the risk of default. Also, to the extent that such programs differentially subsidize debt over equity (Cromwell et al., 1984), they have effects analogous to cost-based systems.

III. DATA SOURCES

Data for this analysis are drawn from the 1983 Capital Finance Survey, the 1982 Annual Survey of Hospitals, and the 1983 Multihospital System Validation Survey. Each of these surveys was conducted by the AHA. Means and standard deviations of the variables used in the multivariate analyses are found in Appendix Table A–1.

The Capital Finance Survey (CFS) consisted of a mail questionnaire sent to all short-term, general acute care hospitals. In addition to obtaining information on the hospital's balance sheet and income statements, the survey included detailed questions concerning all outstanding hospital debt: type and amounts of issue, the amounts repaid at the time of the survey, and the most recent hospital bond rating. The survey had 2768 respondents, yielding a response rate of 47.9%. Although this is a low response rate by AHA standards, the pattern of response is typical of most AHA special-topic surveys (Mullner et al., 1981). Hospitals that are investor-owned, small, rural, or in the South are underrepresented. Of particular significance, relatively few members of large investor-owned chains responded to the survey. As a consequence, the investor-owned chain hospital respondents mainly belonged to small chains.

Unfortunately, the CFS did not obtain information on the year the debt was issued. To estimate the year, we employed two alternative assumptions: (1) a constant amount of principal is paid off each year; (2) the sum of annual interest and principal repayments is constant. The first assumption resulted in more plausible issue dates (a higher correlation between the debt yield and the federal funds rate for the "issue year" and less erratic variation in the rates). Results presented in this study are based on the first assumption.

The Annual Survey of Hospitals was sent to all U.S. hospitals. In 1982, the response rate was 91%. This survey provided data on hospital ownership, sources of revenue, and information needed to construct financial ratios. Underrepresentation, therefore, is far less of a problem with Annual

Survey of Hospitals than with CFS data. Yet for certain items, missing values are a problem.

The Validation Survey is a telephone survey of multihospital systems. It provided an identification of those hospitals that were owned, leased, sponsored, or contract-managed by another organization and the effective date of the affiliation.

The issue of representativeness is critical to this study and is of concern, given the relatively low response rate to the Capital Finance Survey. To address this question, we estimated an interest rate equation using Annual Survey of Hospitals data. The dependent variable was hospital interest payment divided by hospital outstanding debt. For each ownership-system-type variable, we included an interaction term taking the value one if the hospital did not respond to the CFS. (See Appendix Table A–2). Throughout this study, we defined a chain hospital as one owned, leased, or sponsored by an outside organization. Hospitals under management contract were considered separately. Further, we distinguished between chain and contract-managed hospitals on the basis of length of the hospital's affiliation with the chain or management firm. A "new" chain or management contract hospital was one affiliated since the beginning of 1979. Other chain and contract-managed hospitals were classified as "old chain" or "old contract-managed." The ownership category of the contract-managed hospitals is that of the hospital. The CFS respondents were comparable to Annual Survey respondents with respect to interest rate paid with one exception: independent government nonrespondents to the CFS paid statistically significantly higher interest rates than respondents in this system status–ownership group. However, to the extent that large investor-owned chain hospitals, for example, do not respond to the AHA Annual Survey, then our results may not be generalizable.

IV.   DESCRIPTIVE EVIDENCE

A.   Debt

Frequency distributions of sources of hospital debt, based on 4124 active debt issues as of 1983, are shown in Table 1. The sources are direct loan, taxable bond, tax-exempt bond, lease, and other debt. In performing the calculations, we weighted by the face value of the loan.

Several patterns are consistent with conventional wisdom. First, private nonprofit hospitals, whether independent or system, obtained most of their debt from tax-exempt bonds. Tax-exempt debt constituted 69–82% of the debt incurred after 1978. The move to tax-exempt financing appears to have accelerated in the late 1970s, particularly for chain hospitals. This finding is consistent with Metz (1983), who reported that the dollar amount

Table 1. Percentage of Hospital Debt From Various Sources, 1983

Hospital	Year of Issue	Direct Loan	Taxable Bond	Tax-Exempt Bond	Lease	Other
Nonprofit						
Independent	Pre-1973	28.4	4.3*	47.2	13.5	6.7
	1973–1978	26.3	7.0	57.1	5.2	4.4
	Post-1978	19.1	3.1	68.9	3.5	5.4
Old Chain	Pre-1973	15.7	6.0*	56.5	21.2	0.6
	1973–1978	37.8	13.7	38.4	8.2	1.9
	Post-1978	15.9	5.6	74.8	1.6	2.1
New Chain	Pre-1973	37.6*	5.2*	36.3*	17.2*	3.7
	1973–1978	52.1	5.3*	11.9*	27.6	3.1*
	Post-1978	12.4	3.4*	82.4	1.0	0.9
Investor-owned						
Independent	Pre-1973	97.8*	0.0	0.0	2.2*	0.0
	1973–1978	99.8*	0.0	0.0	0.2*	0.0
	Post-1978	72.3	0.0	8.6*	19.1	0.1*
Chain	Pre-1973	0.0	0.0	0.0	0.0	0.0
	1973–1978	58.8*	0.0	0.0	41.2*	0.0
	Post-1978	87.1	0.0	0.0	12.9*	0.0
Government						
Independent	Pre-1973	1.5	0.6*	70.6	24.7	2.5*
	1973–1978	6.5	4.6*	70.7	7.3	10.9
	Post-1978	3.5	1.6*	73.8	8.5	12.6
Chain	Pre-1973	35.3*	0.0	10.5*	54.2*	0.0
	1973–1978	12.8*	0.0	87.2*	0.0	0.0
	Post-1978	21.5	0.0	71.8*	0.2*	6.5*
Contract-Managed by—						
Nonprofit						
Old	Pre-1973	15.7	6.0*	56.5	21.2	0.6
	1973–1978	37.8	13.7	38.4	8.2	1.9
	Post-1978	15.9	5.6	74.8	1.6	2.1
New	Pre-1973	30.2*	51.4*	1.0*	16.9*	0.6*
	1973–1978	48.0	0.0	39.4*	11.7	0.9*
	Post-1978	23.3	5.6*	68.1	2.3	0.8*
Investor-Owned						
Old	Pre-1973	76.0*	0.0	0.0	24.0*	0.0
	1973–1978	29.9	0.0	66.8*	3.3	0.0
	Post-1978	20.9	5.3*	73.3	0.5*	0.0
New	Pre-1973	4.1*	0.0	40.9*	17.1*	38.0*
Contract	1973–1978	6.2	2.4*	65.0	18.6	7.7
	Post-1978	8.1	1.3*	85.1	2.8	2.8

Note: *Cell includes fewer than five observations.
Source: Unpublished data from American Hospital Association, Capital Finance Survey, 1983.

of tax-exempt bond issues increased over 73% between 1976 and 1977. The change primarily reflected a shift from direct loans and leases. System hospitals have relied more extensively on tax-exempt debt than have independent hospitals. This may reflect the transactions costs arguments noted above.

As with private nonprofit facilities, system status made little difference in source of debt for investor-owned hospitals. Direct loans and private placements have dominated. These patterns would probably have differed if the CFS sample had included hospital members of larger investor-owned chains. Government facilities were similar to their private nonprofit counterparts in relying on tax-exempt debt. This is consistent with hospital construction survey data (Metz, 1983). However, government institutions were more likely to use "other debt sources" than were other hospitals in our sample.

Finally, contract-managed hospitals, whether managed by investor-owned or nonprofit systems, had similar sources of debt. The distribution of sources tended to reflect the pattern of independent nonprofit hospitals. This finding is plausible for two reasons. First, most contract-managed hospitals are independent nonprofit (Morrisey and Alexander, 1985). Second, the management contract does not allow all of the pooling and transactions cost reductions available to fully integrated systems.

B. Bond Ratings

Distributions of bond ratings by hospital ownership and system status are shown in Table 2. Unfortunately, the time frame in which these ratings were received is not well grounded. Each hospital was only asked in 1983 to report its most recent bond rating. Nevertheless, the ratings in Table 2 are generally consistent with earlier studies reported by Ermann and Gabel (1984). The private nonprofit and government systems hospitals had a larger proportion of bonds ranked in the "A" categories than did their independent counterparts. Further, the independent and contract-managed hospitals were much more likely not to have a debt rating.

It is dangerous to infer from this comparison that system hospitals have lower costs of debt capital. First, bond ratings are based upon quantitative and qualitative determinations of the rating firm. These factors are said to include financial and medical staff variables, hospital market conditions, as well as management and legal factors (Booz, Allen, and Hamilton, 1983). No prior study has controlled for other factors when assessing the relationship between "systemness" and bond rating. Second, there is no empirical evidence for the hospital industry on the responsiveness of cost of debt to changes in bond ratings. Thompson (1986, pp. 4–5) reported that the spread in municipal bond yields rated Baa to those rated A by

Table 2. Percentage of Hospitals With Various Bond Ratings, Recent Years

Hospital Type	AAA	A+ to AA	A to A−	BBB+ to BBB−	BB+ to D−	Provisional A− to AAA	Provisional B to BBB+	Unavailable	Not Rated
Nonprofit									
Independent	2.4	10.4	22.4	3.4	0.7	3.4	0.8	13.3	43.2
Old Chain	1.9	25.0	19.9	2.7	0.0	6.3	0.2	12.9	31.1
New Chain	3.8	24.4	21.8	1.3	0.0	0.0	2.6	19.2	26.9
Investor-owned									
Independent	0.0	0.0	0.0	0.0	0.0	0.0	0.0	6.2	93.8
Chain	0.0	0.0	0.0	0.0	0.0	0.0	0.0	0.0	100.0
Government									
Independent	1.9	7.1	16.4	4.6	0.0	4.6	0.6	23.9	40.9
Chain	45.4	18.2	0.0	0.0	0.0	0.0	0.0	0.0	36.4
Contract-Managed by—									
Nonprofit									
Old	0.0	7.9	15.8	2.6	0.0	2.6	0.0	31.6	39.5
New	13.8	3.9	7.8	7.8	5.9	0.0	2.0	23.5	35.3
Investor-Owned									
Old	0.0	0.0	20.0	10.0	0.0	3.3	6.7	3.3	56.7
New	4.3	1.4	8.6	5.7	1.4	0.0	0.0	35.7	42.9

Source: Unpublished data from American Hospital Association, Capital Finance Survey, 1983.

calendar quarter for the years 1980–1985 ranged from 15 to 92 basis points; the spread between Baa and Aa bond yields ranged from 36 to 148 basis points during this period. There is evidence that the cost of debt is relatively insensitive to bond ratings. Ederington et al. (1984, p. 19), concluded that, after controlling for publicly available financial data on a sample of U.S. firms, the difference in yield between a Moody's Baa and Ba rating, for example, was only 37 basis points.

Finally, according to conventional wisdom, hospitals without bond ratings must pay a higher price for debt. However, the ability to predict bond ratings is well known. Kaplan and Urwitz (1979, p. 265), for example, concluded that "a simple model . . . can correctly classify about two-thirds of a holdout sample of newly issued bonds. . . . No bond is predicted more than one rating category away [from its true rating]." Thus, unrated hospitals may face only slightly higher costs of debt if holders can relatively easily determine the degree of risk involved.

C.   Financial Status

Since bond ratings in particular, and the cost of capital to hospitals more generally, depend on standard accounting ratios, we examined several ratios by hospital ownership and system status with data from the 1982 Annual Survey of Hospitals (Table 3). We constructed the ratios by summing values from individual hospitals to derive numerators and denominators of a ratio before dividing. Thus, larger hospitals received a larger weight, thereby keeping extreme values from small hospitals from disproportionately influencing the estimated ratios.

Current assets divided by current liabilities, the current ratio, is a measure of hospital liquidity, i.e., the ability to meet short-term debt obligations. The sample mean was 2.00, but the mean ratio varied appreciably by ownership and system status. Surprisingly, independent hospitals had the highest ratios. Their chain counterparts had the lowest ratios. This may be a reflection of the chains' ability to hold and invest cash from the corporate office.

Days in receivable measures effectiveness of management in minimizing unproductive financial assets. Receivables per se provide no revenue to the hospital. The industry mean in 1982 was 65 days. Government hospitals performed quite badly in this dimension. It is tempting to attribute this to heavier bad debt/charity loads. However, metropolitan and nonmetropolitan public hospitals overall had only 8.6% and 5.3% of gross patient revenue attributable to bad debt and charity, respectively, in 1982; the latter figure in particular, was only slightly above the industry averages (Sloan et al., 1986, p. 23).

The ratio of short-term to total debt provides some indication of how the hospitals structure their portfolios of debt. Too much reliance on short-

Table 3. Financial Ratios by Hospital Ownership and Chain Status, 1982

	N	Current Ratio	Days In Receivables	Short-Term Debt/Total Debt	Debt/Equity	Return on Equity	Total Margin
All Hospitals	4,103	2.00	65.2	0.29	0.79	0.075	0.043
Nonprofit							
Independent	1,973	1.92	62.3	0.29	0.79	0.071	0.042
Old Chain	510	1.95	61.3	0.27	0.92	0.096	0.051
New Chain	96	1.91	61.8	0.26	1.06	0.111	0.053
Old Mgt. Contract	57	1.90	69.4	0.32	0.76	0.091	0.051
New Mgt. Contract	95	1.84	67.4	0.24	1.13	0.080	0.041
Investor-owned							
Independent	98	1.77	70.4	0.35	2.24	0.351	0.071
Old Chain	48	2.25	63.5	0.33	0.99	0.338	0.113
New Chain	33	2.20	66.2	0.19	1.61	0.163	0.061
Old Mgt. Contract	35	2.02	58.8	0.19	1.53	0.109	0.048
New Mgt. Contract	138	1.82	64.9	0.28	0.89	0.048	0.028
Government							
Independent	992	2.56	79.0	0.36	0.50	0.056	0.030
Chain	24	1.60	113.0	0.64	0.66	-0.016	-0.0073

Source: Unpublished data from American Hospital Association, Annual Hospital Survey, 1982.

term (less than a year) instruments tends to be risky. Overall, the industry had 29% of its debt in short-term debt. Government and independent investor-owned hospitals were most dependent on short-term debt.

Overall, the debt-to-equity ratio was 0.79 in 1982. We measured equity in book value (the hospital's fund balance). Independent for-profit hospitals were almost three times as levered as the industry. Established systems were more highly levered than the industry as a whole. Although above the industry average, investor-owned system hospitals had a lower debt-to-equity ratio than their independent counterparts. The estimated debt-to-equity ratios for investor-owned chains reported in Table 3 are reasonably similar to estimates based on company balance sheet data (Valvona and Sloan, 1985).

Return on equity (ROE) in 1982 was 7.5% for the hospital industry as a whole. Private nonprofit hospitals did half again as well as government institutions. However, independent and old-chain investor-owned hospitals had ROEs over 33%.

The final column of Table 3 provides a measure of operating surplus. If we examine the nonprofit sector, we find that operating profits were fairly uniform across independent and system hospitals. Differences in "profitability" are attributable to differences in the proportion of debt carried by the various nonprofit hospital groups. Old-chain investor-owned hospitals had margins well above the industry average.

The investor-owned sector provides a study in contrasts. First, relative to nonprofit freestanding hospitals, independent investor-owned hospitals had higher margins, almost 70% more surplus for each dollar of revenue. However, the major reason for their higher return on equity resulted from their being more highly levered. Their debt-to-equity ratio was almost three times that of the freestanding private nonprofits. The high return on equity for long-time chain hospitals vis-à-vis nonprofit chain hospitals arose almost exclusively from differences in margins. Their debt-to-equity ratio was about equal to the nonprofit hospitals'.

V. REGRESSION ANALYSIS

A. Bond Ratings

There is a growing literature in finance and accounting on determinants of bond ratings (Fisher, 1959; Horrigan, 1966; West, 1970; Pinches and Minger, 1973; Kaplan and Urwitz, 1979). These studies have generally examined financial characteristics of the firm as well as characteristics of the debt. Our research on bond ratings departed from tradition in two ways. First, we did not have data on variability of hospital earnings; nor did we know whether particular debt issues were subordinated. Second, unlike the more general empirical investigations, we included measures of the external environment, mandatory rate regulation and cost-based payment programs, and measures of ownership and system status.

Because bond ratings refer to discrete, mutually exclusive categories, we employed multinominal logit analysis. To keep the number of categories manageable, we combined ratings into four categories: unavailable or not rated; provisional rating; ratings BBB to D; and ratings above BBB. Ratings above BBB were the excluded category.

Coefficients for ownership and system status are statistically insignificant with several exceptions (Table 4). Private nonprofit chains were more likely to be rated and, when rated, more likely to have ratings in the A range than were independent government hospitals, the omitted reference category. Government chain hospitals tended to have higher ratings. Many of the contract-managed hospitals, both nonprofit and investor-owned, had ratings in the BBB + to D − range. A number of coefficients on the system variables have high associated standard errors. This is due to zero or a very small number of observations in the cell.

Within ownership categories, chain hospitals were more likely to be rated than independent hospitals, even controlling for financial characteristics. This may be a reflection of the volume of debt floated by chains. If the desired debt issue is too large to be easily handled through direct loans and private placements, systems may be forced to obtain ratings to enter the public market.

Financial characteristics of the hospital provide a better explanation of the hospital's bond rating than system affiliation or ownership. Successful operating performance measured by total margin was associated with both being rated and having higher bond ratings. However, greater leverage was likely to result in a low or no rating, but had no effect on the likelihood of a provisional rating. While the debt load of an institution is of major concern to a lender, changes in the debt-to-equity ratio were probably foreshadowed by other events that warranted the provisional rating. Hospitals in relatively liquid positions, measured by higher current ratios, and those with more short-term relative to long-term debt were more likely to be unrated and particularly unlikely to have provisional ratings. Hospitals with lots of short-term debt probably relied more on direct loans.

Days in receivable and the percentage of gross revenue considered to be charity care or bad debt had statistically insignificant effects on bond ratings. However, changes in these measures apparently serve as signals of deteriorating financial position since they were positively related to receiving a provisional rating.

Coefficients on third-party reimbursement variables are generally insignificant. Hospital dependence on revenue from cost-based sources had essentially no effects on ratings. The presence of a mandatory rate-setting

Table 4. Bond Ratings Regressions

Explanatory Variables	Not Available/ Not Rated	BBB+ to D− Rating	Provisional Rating
Constant	−1.333***	−2.457***	−1.016
	(0.285)	(0.816)	(0.668)
Nonprofit, Independent	−0.170	0.084	−0.169
	(0.149)	(0.438)	(0.300)
Nonprofit, Old Chain	−0.536***	−1.878**	0.008
	(0.179)	(0.816)	(0.340)
Nonprofit, New Chain	−0.798***	−13.642	−1.205
	(0.303)	(333.504)	(0.782)
Nonprofit, Old Contract-Managed	−0.039	0.602	−0.175
	(0.477)	(1.133)	(1.100)
Nonprofit, New Contract-Managed	0.309	2.362***	−0.621
	(0.434)	(0.632)	(1.088)
Investor-Owned, Independent	16.463	2.261	1.990
	(1100.8)	(1705.2)	(1617.33)
Investor-Owned, Chain	15.891	2.399	2.192
	(1027.12)	(1736.31)	(1680.59)
Investor-Owned, Old Contract-Managed	0.323	2.039**	1.272
	(0.580)	(0.827)	(0.774)
Investor-Owned, New Contract-Managed	1.310***	1.484*	−13.469
	(0.378)	(0.760)	(369.399)
Government, Chain	−2.795***	−13.137	−14.126
	(0.751)	(881.144)	(924.171)
Return on Equity	0.616	−0.008	−0.203
	(0.473)	(0.872)	(1.024)
Total Margin	−11.491***	−2.518	−3.296
	(1.720)	(4.051)	(3.819)
Days in Receivable	−0.004	0.001	0.029***
	(0.003)	(0.009)	(0.006)
Current Ratio	0.266***	0.095	−0.806***
	(0.040)	(0.109)	(0.167)
Percent Bad Debt and Charity	−0.644	−8.656	5.076**
	(1.576)	(6.051)	(2.413)
Debt/Equity	0.067**	0.085**	−0.022
	(0.027)	(0.041)	(0.064)
Short-term/Total Debt	5.668***	−1.041	−4.414***
	(0.355)	(1.221)	(1.121)
Percent Cost Based	0.119	−0.240	−0.246
	(0.191)	(0.524)	(0.402)
Rate Setting	0.325**	0.360	−0.307
	(0.138)	(0.376)	(0.323)

*Significant at the 10% level, two-tail test.
**Significant at the 5% level, two-tail test.
***Significant at the 1% level, two-tail test.

program was somewhat more likely to result in lower bond ratings, but more importantly, hospitals in states with mandatory rate-setting programs were significantly less likely to be rated.

B. Hospital Debt Yields

We estimated two regressions with CFS data (Table 5). The first is limited to 2655 debt issues obtained by hospitals between 1979 and 1983, with a mean yield of 10.38%. The second includes the 4125 debt instruments issued since 1940 which were still outstanding in 1983. The mean yield for this sample is 9.72%.

We first controlled for the life of the debt instrument and the federal funds rate at the time the debt was issued. Relative to debt of less than 10 years, longer-term debt had a lower yield. Term structures are generally explained by consideration of a liquidity preference and inflationary expectations (Copeland and Weston, 1984). The liquidity preference implies that a longer-term debt is riskier. The expectations theory holds that, in addition, the term structure will reflect the market's perceptions of future inflation. Our results suggest that the market was anticipating lower future inflation than when the bonds were issued; a survey conducted at another time with different inflationary expectations could have revealed the opposite.

The federal funds rate measures the level of nominal interest rates when the bond was issued. During 1979–1983, a 1% increase in the federal funds rate increased the yield on new hospital debt by one-third of 1%.

Several variables account for the effect of type of debt on yield. Relative to direct loans, the excluded category, tax-exempt bonds were 1.08 and 1.31 interest points lower for recent and all debt, respectively. This reflects the tax avoidance potential for bondholders. In theory, leases are perfect substitutes for debt. Their advantage generally stems from their tax savings potential. If one party to the lease has a higher marginal tax rate than the other, the lease offers a vehicle to transfer tax savings from the lower-taxed firm to the higher. The low-tax firm is compensated through an adjustment in the lease fee. Given the differential tax treatment, a plausible match is a nonprofit lease from a for-profit leasor. Judging from the Table 5 regressions, leasing appears to be an expensive form of debt, more expensive than any other debt instrument.

Surprisingly, private nonprofit independent hospitals had virtually the same cost of debt as did established nonprofit system-owned hospitals; both exceeded independent government hospital cost of debt, the omitted reference group, by about 1.4%. Independent nonprofit hospitals had lower debt costs than did more recently acquired nonprofit system hospitals. This finding must be interpreted with caution, however. The result was obtained

Table 5.   Yield on Debt Regressions (Standard Errors in Parentheses)

Explanatory Variables	Recent Issue (Issue Year > 1978)	All Issues (Issue Year > 1939)
Constant	3.077***	4.617***
	(0.784)	(0.475)
Life 10–19 Years	−1.638***	−1.236***
	(0.162)	(0.123)
Life 20–29 Years	−2.292***	−1.931***
	(0.166)	(0.139)
Life 30+ Years	−1.828***	−2.039***
	(0.267)	(0.209)
Federal Funds Rate	0.363***	0.280***
	(0.047)	(0.016)
Taxable Bond	−0.172	−0.363
	(0.336)	(0.270)
Tax-Exempt Bond	−1.084***	−1.312***
	(0.158)	(0.129)
Lease	2.420***	2.571***
	(0.159)	(0.126)
Other Debt	0.114	0.143
	(0.208)	(0.167)
Nonprofit, Independent	1.474***	1.394***
	(0.166)	(0.134)
Nonprofit, Old Chain	1.401***	1.365***
	(0.208)	(0.168)
Nonprofit, New Chain	1.659***	1.202***
	(0.362)	(0.295)
Nonprofit, Old Mgt. Contract	1.239**	1.115***
	(0.486)	(0.377)
Nonprofit, New Mgt. Contract	1.917***	1.438***
	(0.433)	(0.335)
Investor-Owned, Independent	1.821**	1.919***
	(0.741)	(0.672)
Investor-Owned, Chain	4.368***	4.233***
	(0.940)	(0.804)
Investor-Owned, Old Mgt. Contract	3.626***	4.159***
	(0.553)	(0.440)
Investor-Owned, New Mgt. Contract	1.391***	0.672**
	(0.370)	(0.286)
Government, Chain	1.670*	0.810
	(0.898)	(0.650)
AA to AA+ Rating	1.030**	0.783**
	(0.432)	(0.356)
A+ Rating	0.908**	0.427
	(0.416)	(0.338)

Table 5. (continued)

Explanatory Variables	Recent Issue (Issue Year > 1978)	All Issues (Issue Year > 1939)
A − to A Rating	0.930**	0.553*
	(0.373)	(0.310)
BBB + Rating	0.786	0.397
	(0.547)	(0.465)
BBB − to BBB Rating	0.824	0.563
	(0.540)	(0.427)
D to BB + Rating	1.537*	1.230
	(0.845)	(0.833)
Provisional A to AAA Rating	1.413***	1.083***
	(0.455)	(0.381)
Provisional B to BBB +	1.660**	1.235*
	(0.723)	(0.635)
Rating Not Available	0.847**	0.560*
	(0.380)	(0.313)
Not Rated	1.004***	0.599**
	(0.366)	(0.302)
Total Margin	0.207	1.459
	(1.330)	(1.058)
Debt/Equity	0.238***	0.251***
	(0.055)	(0.047)
(Debt/Equity)squared	−0.007***	−0.007***
	(0.002)	(0.002)
Days In receivable	−0.002	−0.001
	(0.003)	(0.003)
Current Ratio	0.062*	0.062***
	(0.033)	(0.023)
Short-term/Long-term Debt	1.602***	1.479***
	(0.332)	(0.262)
Percent Bad Debt & Charity	0.384	− 0.261
	(1.711)	(1.389)
Percent Cost Based	1.006**	0.608*
	(0.430)	(0.359)
Rate Setting	0.219	0.134
	(0.159)	(0.128)
R^2	0.39	0.40
$\bar{R}^2$	0.38	0.39
Observations	2755	4125

Notes: *Significant at the 10%, two-tail test.
 **Significant at the 5%, two-tail test.
 ***Significant at the 1%, two-tail test.

by controlling for a variety of factors, including the riskiness of the institution. Thus, the finding implies that there are factors not associated with our measures of risk that enable independent nonprofit hospitals to attract low-cost debt. Since many of the independent nonprofit hospitals are not rated by bond agencies, it may be that many unrated hospitals are low-risk institutions fully capable of obtaining direct loans and private placements at favorable rates.

The same lower cost relationship between independent and system-owned hospitals is found in the parameters for proprietary hospitals. The independent institutions attracted debt—from whatever source—at a rate of 2.5 percentage points lower than the investor-owned chains in our sample. Again, one must be cautious in this comparison, since hospitals in large investor-owned chains did not generally respond to the CFS.

Comparisons between investor-owned and nonprofit debt yields indicate that independent investor-owned facilities faced debt costs about a quarter of a point above those of private nonprofit facilities. On the other hand, investor-owned chain hospitals faced a cost of debt approximately 3.0 points above that of established nonprofit chain hospitals. These differences largely reflect the payment of income taxes by the for-profit organizations. Since we controlled for risk and source of debt (particularly tax-exempt debt), yields should be equal across firms except for tax payment differences.

Relative yields of contract-managed hospitals were generally lower than the yields of investor-owned chain hospitals. The differences may reflect the mix of tax-paying and tax-exempt facilities, but also the investor-owned chains in the CFS sample were small and not representative of investor-owned chains in general.

To address the issue of hospital risk, we included the most recent bond ratings of the hospital and selected financial ratios. As anticipated, hospitals with ratings under AAA had a higher cost of debt capital. However, relationship between ratings and yields is not monotonic. This may reflect the relatively small number of ratings in some cells. For recent issues, ratings between BBB − and AA + add 1 point to the yield on debt. Ratings below BBB − add about 1½ points.[2]

Provisional ratings generally reflect the intention of the rating agency to lower the bond rating of the institution. Thus, such ratings plausibly imply higher yields. The size of the coefficients generally exceed the worst-case rating, however. This can perhaps be explained by the nature of our data. The yield data include issues 1979–1983 and 1940–1983, while the bond ratings are "the most recent." Thus, there is measurement error. Since provisional ratings are temporary and subject to change, it is likely that they are more contemporaneous with the yield values. The bond rating coefficients are more likely to be understated than the provisional rates are to be overstated. Analogously, we are more likely to have underestimated the D to BB+ rating than we are to have overstated the provisional rating.

We also included "rating not available" and "hospital not rated" variables to reflect the large numbers of hospitals without formal bond ratings. The results suggest that while these hospitals are riskier than AAA-rated hospitals, they only pay 1 point of interest more. Thus, their cost of debt is comparable to the vast majority of rated hospitals.

Even though individual bond rating coefficients are statistically significant, we cannot reject the null hypothesis that they do not affect the yield on hospital debt as a group. That is, the remaining variables in the regression do as good a job in predicting bond yield as is done by the larger set including bond rating. This adds further evidence to the case that unrated hospitals are not necessarily disadvantaged in the capital market.

The financial ratios do not perform as robustly as anticipated. We would expect improvements in total margin, the hospital performance from operations, to reduce its cost of debt. The results are small in absolute value, of the wrong sign, and statistically insignificant, suggesting that total margin has no effect on hospital cost of debt, controlling for bond ratings, which are affected by margins and other factors.

The debt-to-equity ratio does imply higher cost of debt with greater hospital debt. We included a squared term to ascertain whether the marginal effect of indebtedness on the cost of debt capital increases with the amount of indebtedness. The negative sign on the coefficients of the squared term does not support this shape. For small and moderate changes in the debt-to-equity ratio, the squared term only subtracts a little.

The coefficients on the current ratio suggest that the ability to cover short-term obligations is associated with higher costs of debt. It may be that the market perceives hospitals as holding too much cash and views this as indicating less than prudent management. A higher proportion of short-term debt is associated with higher yields as anticipated, as is a higher bad debt and charity load.

Finally, we examined the effects of payment policies on the cost of debt. The yield increased with the proportion of patient revenue coming from cost-based sources. As indicated above, cost-based payment systems reduce the risk and subsidize the use of debt for nonprofit organizations. These debt-cost-reducing factors could have been offset by cost-containment actions that reduced payments to hospitals. Or, since hospitals with high shares of revenue from cost-based sources could shift a large part of interest expense on to third-party payers, they had less of an incentive to search for low-cost debt. From our analysis, it is apparent that the interest payment guarantee effect of cost-based payment dominated.

Rate-setting programs were expected to increase capital costs by restricting payment levels. Our results suggest that mandatory state-run programs increased hospital debt costs by a fifth of a percentage point on average in recent years. The result, however, lacks statistical significance. Rate-setting also affected the likelihood that the hospital had a bond rating, and unrated hospitals did pay slightly more for debt. So there is a small indirect effect of rate setting on the cost of debt.

VI.   DISCUSSION AND IMPLICATIONS

We began this study with a series of nine questions concerning the cost of debt capital to the hospital industry. On the basis of our analysis, we offer the following answers:

1.   Investor-owned hospitals, both chain-owned and independent, generated more revenue from operations and were more highly levered than were nonprofit hospitals. As a consequence, they had higher returns on equity.

2.   Hospitals differed by ownership in sources of debt capital. Investor-owned firms relied on direct loans primarily, while nonprofit firms used tax-exempt bond financing extensively. The use of the debt instruments expanded in the late 1970s.

3.   The cost of debt capital was much higher for investor-owned than for nonprofit hospitals, whether system-owned or independent. This difference is largely attributable to the tax status of investor-owned hospitals. It is also the case, however, that independent investor-owned hospitals faced somewhat lower debt costs than did system-owned hospitals. Nonprofit hospitals faced almost identical debt costs, irrespective of chain status.

4.   Relative to direct loans, taxable and tax-exempt bonds as well as leases became less expensive over time. However, recently issued taxable bonds were still 18 basis points (0.18 of 1% of interest) and tax-exempt bonds 108 basis points below direct loans when measured on yield. Leases were the most expensive form of debt.

5.   In general, lower bond ratings raised the cost of capital. The effects were relatively small, however. A rating in the range BB+ to D raised the yield on debt by only about 120 to 150 basis points relative to AAA ratings. Provisional ratings had similar effects. Being unrated raised yield rates by no more than 1 percentage point.

6.   Our results suggest that differences in bond ratings have more to do with the characteristics of the organizations than with system or ownership status. System affiliation did not affect bond ratings directly but may do so by systematic management efforts to affect institutional riskiness.

7.   While the theoretical finance literature is divided on the effects of the debt-to-equity ratio on the cost of capital, our data suggest that

it has a small effect on the yield on hospital debt. Evaluated at the observational means, an increase in the ratio of 0.10 increased the cost of debt by 2 basis points.

8. Hospital dependence on cost-based reimbursement raised the cost of debt capital. Any favorable effect of cost-based reimbursement on hospital credit risk appears to be more than offset by other factors, such as reduced incentive to secure low-interest rate loans.

9. If anything, rate-setting programs increased the cost of debt, but only by a small amount.

The "big picture" question that caused us to undertake this study was whether system hospitals truly face advantages in capital markets and consequently have grown relative to their independent counterparts. Our results on the whole suggest that system status per se has been overemphasized, at least as far as the cost of debt capital is concerned. The share of interest expense in total expense is simply too small (less than 5% on average, from unpublished tabulations of Annual Survey of Hospitals data), and the effect of "systemness" on debt yields too small for the cost of debt per se to be a major reason for joining a system.

There are four possible criticisms of our conclusion, and we shall examine each in turn:

First, our sample is unrepresentative. Although the sample is unrepresentative in ways noted above, we have performed various cross-checks. The unrepresentative feature that concerns us most is the nature of the investor-owned chain hospital respondents to the Capital Finance Survey. Hospital members of large investor-owned chains are underrepresented. One can be sure that sources of debt capital for large investor-owned chain hospitals differ, and it is possible, if not likely, that their cost of debt capital is lower as well. Investor-owned hospital respondents to the Annual Survey of Hospitals are somewhat more representative, and key financial ratios reported in Table 3 are consistent with those reported by the largest 10 chains in their annual 10-K reports.

Second, the system hospitals may not show a lower cost of debt capital because those hospitals facing a high cost of capital joined systems. The split of system and contract-managed hospitals on "old" vs. "new" was an attempt to circumvent this potential selectivity problem. Certainly by the time a hospital becomes an "old" system member or an "old" management contract hospital, it should no longer have poor access to debt capital. Yet the coefficients on the "old" system and contract variables were not that different from their new counterparts.

Third, we used the hospital as the observational unit. Particularly for investor-owned chains and to a much lesser extent for nonprofit chains, one could argue for using the system as the more appropriate unit. To check the sensitivity of our results, we reestimated the bond rating and yield equations with data limited to the nonsystem hospitals. The regression coefficients and associated standard errors were very close to the findings reported in Tables 4 and 5.

Fourth, the rationale for joining a chain may have more to do with access to equity than to debt capital. This point, which has merit, only applies to investor-owned chains. Yet, although publicly held investor-owned hospitals have an important advantage in the sale of equity, it is not at all clear why their debt-to-equity ratios are far higher than those in the nonprofit hospital sector (Valvona and Sloan, 1985). Furthermore, if a firm in general and a hospital in particular can sell both debt and equity securities, the cost of each will be equal at the margin. Thus, an institution with a high price of debt also pays a high price for equity. Resolving this and other related puzzles represents a challenge for future research.

APPENDIX

Table A-1. Means and Standards Deviations

Explanatory Variables	Recent Issues Equation	All issues Equation
Yield	10.38	9.72
	(3.63)	(3.73)
Life 10–19 Years	0.18	0.27
	(0.39)	(0.45)
Life 20–29 Years	0.20	0.20
	(0.40)	(0.40)
Life 30+ Years	0.05	0.06
	(0.23)	(0.24)
Federal Funds Rate	11.84	9.77
	(1.20)	(3.05)
Taxable Bond	0.03	0.03
	(0.18)	(0.18)
Tax-Exempt Bond	0.31	0.28
	(0.46)	(0.45)
Lease	0.22	0.24
	(0.42)	(0.42)
Other Debt	0.09	0.10
	(0.29)	(0.29)
Nonprofit, Independent	0.55	0.53
	(0.50)	(0.50)
Nonprofit, Old Chain	0.16	0.15
	(0.36)	(0.36)
Nonprofit, New Chain	0.03	0.03
	(0.17)	(0.17)

Table A-1. (continued)

Explanatory Variables	Recent Issues Equation	All issues Equation
Nonprofit, Old Mgt. Contract	0.01 (0.12)	0.02 (0.13)
Nonprofit, New Mgt. Contract	0.02 (0.14)	0.02 (0.14)
Investor-Owned, Independent	0.006 (0.08)	0.005 (0.07)
Investor-Owned, Chain	0.004 (0.06)	0.003 (0.06)
Investor-Owned, Old Mgt. Contract	0.01 (0.11)	0.01 (0.11)
Investor-Owned, New Mgt. Contract	0.03 (0.16)	0.03 (0.17)
Government Chain	0.004 (0.06)	0.005 (0.07)
AA to AA+ Rating	0.05 (0.23)	0.05 (0.22)
A+ Rating	0.06 (0.25)	0.07 (0.25)
A− to A Rating	0.20 (0.40)	0.18 (0.39)
BBB+ Rating	0.02 (0.13)	0.02 (0.12)
BBB− to BBB Rating	0.02 (0.13)	0.02 (0.14)
D to BB+ Rating	0.005 (0.07)	0.003 (0.06)
Provisional A− to AAA	0.04 (0.19)	0.03 (0.18)
Provisional B to BBB+	0.008 (0.09)	0.007 (0.08)
Not Available	0.16 (0.37)	0.17 (0.38)
Not Rated	0.41 (0.49)	0.42 (0.49)
Total Margin	0.04 (0.05)	0.04 (0.05)
Debt/Equity	1.53 (2.15)	1.42 (1.92)
(Debt/Equity)squared	6.97 (59.11)	5.72 (47.97)
Days in Receivables	63.13 (19.04)	62.82 (18.64)

(*continued*)

Table A-1.   (continued)

Explanatory Variables	Recent Issues Equation	All issues Equation
Current Ratio	2.36 (1.91)	2.42 (2.17)
Short-term/Long-term Debt	0.34 (0.22)	0.36 (0.23)
Bad Debt and Charity as Percent of Revenue	0.04 (0.04)	0.04 (0.04)
Percent Cost Based	0.50 (0.14)	0.50 (0.14)
Rate Setting	0.16 (0.37)	0.17 (0.38)
Return on Equity	0.08 (0.13)	0.08 (0.13)

Table A-2.   Interest Rate Equation[a]

Explanatory Variables	Mean Value	Coefficient	Std. Error
Dependent Variable	0.054		
Constant	—	0.052***	0.002
Nonrespondent CFS	0.037	0.025*	0.014
Nonprofit	0.524	0.004***	0.001
Nonrespondent CFS	0.021	−0.014	0.014
Nonprofit Old Chain	0.143	0.005***	0.002
Nonrespondent CFS	0.001	−0.005	0.019
Nonprofit New Chain	0.027	0.006*	0.003
Nonrespondent CFS	0.0003	−0.020	0.027
Nonprofit Old Contract Mgt.	0.011	−0.002	0.004
Nonprofit New Contract Mgt.	0.023	0.005	0.003
Investor-Owned	0.026	0.019***	0.004
Nonrespondent CFS	0.010	−0.023	0.015
Investor-Owned Chain	0.022	0.014***	0.004
Nonrespondent CFS	0.003	−0.022	0.017
Investor-Owned Old Contract Mgt.	0.007	0.013**	0.006
Investor-Owned New Contract Mgt.	0.030	0.005	0.003
Government Chain	0.004	0.003	0.007
Nonrespondent CFS	0.0004	−0.043	0.028
Age of Plant	7.611	−0.0001	0.0001
Current Ratio	2.755	0.0006***	0.0002
Days in Receivable (100s)	0.641	−0.003	0.002
Debt/Equity	1.537	0.001***	0.0003
(Debt/Equity)squared	11.739	−0.0000**	0.0000
Return on Equity	0.085	0.001	0.004
Total Margin	0.037	0.003	0.013
Short-term/Long-term Debt	0.360	−0.009***	0.002

Table A-2. Continued

Explanatory Variables	Mean Value	Coefficient	Std. Error
Percent Cost based	0.53	−0.002	0.003
Rate Setting	0.143	−0.002	0.001
R²		0.066	
R̄²		0.057	
Observations		2768	

Notes: ªIf an interact term is missing, it indicates that every hospital in the cell providing the requisite data on the Annual Survey also responded to the CFS.

*Significant at the 10% level, two-tail test.
**Significant at the 5% level, two-tail test.
***Significant at the 1% level, two-tail test.

ACKNOWLEDGMENTS

This study was funded by Grant No. HS–05176 from the National Center for Health Services Research and Health Care Technology Assessment. We are grateful to the Hospital Research and Education Trust for providing access to these data and to Phillip Held, Urban Institute, and Samuel Mitchell, Federation of American Health Systems, for helpful comments on an earlier draft.

NOTES

1. Of course, the finance literature argues that if investors can diversify their portfolios more cheaply than a firm can diversify its products (or locations), then there is no risk reduction from this pooling (see Copeland and Weston, 1984, p. 571–572).
2. The estimates of the effect of risk on yields suffers from a potential selectivity problem which biases the coefficients downward. Systematically excluded from the survey were hospitals which had closed. These hospitals had high risk, ex post. Ex ante their risk measures would have a distribution of values due to measurement error. As to consequence, our risk and yield data disproportionately reflect good risks.

REFERENCES

Alexander, J. A., Lewis, B. L. and Morrisey, M. A. (1985), "Association Strategies of Multihospital Systems." *Health Affairs* 4(3):49–66.
American Hospital Association (1983), *Report of the Special Committee on Equity of Payment for Not-for-Profit and Investor Owned Hospitals.* Chicago: AHA.
Bennett, and Ahrendt (1981), "Achieving Economics of Scale Through Shared Ancillary Services." *Topics in Health Care Financing* 7(3):25–34.
Booz, Allen and Hamilton (1983), "Historical Linkages Between Selected Hospital Characteristics and Bond Ratings." In American Hospital Association, *Report of the Special Committee on Equity of Payment for Not-for-Profit and Investor Owned Hospitals*, Appendix E. Chicago: AHA, May.

Cohodes, D. R. and B. M. Kinkead (1984), *Hospital Capital Formation in the 1980s.* Baltimore: Johns Hopkins University Press.

Conrad, D. A. (1984), "Returns on Equity to Not-for-Profit Decision Making." *Health Services Research* 19(1):41–64.

Copeland, T. E. and Weston, J. F. (1984), *Financial Theory and Corporate Policy*, 2nd ed. Reading, MA: Addison-Wesley.

Cromwell, J., K. A. Colore, and G. Wedig (1984), *Treatment of Capital Cost in Four Medicare-Waivered States: Maryland, New Jersey, New York and Massachusetts.* Washington, DC: U.S. Department of Health and Human Services, Assistant Secretary for Planning and Evaluation, July.

Dorenfest, S. (1981), "Hospital Chains Become Important Providers." *Modern Healthcare* 2(November):77–85.

Ederington, L. H., J. B. Yawitz, and B. E. Roberts (1984), "The Information Content of Bond Ratings." Working paper No. 1323, National Bureau of Economic Research, April.

Ermann, D. and J. Gabel (1984), "Multihospital Systems: Issues and Empirical Findings." *Health Affairs* 3(1):50–64.

Fisher, L. (1959), "Determinanats of Risk Premiums on Corporate Bonds." *Journal of Political Economy* 67:217–37.

Hernandez, M. D. and C. G. Howie (1979), "Capital Financing by Multihospital Systems." In Y. S. Mason (ed.), *Multihospital Arrangements: Public Policy Implications.* Chicago: American Hospital Association, pp. 37–47.

Horrigan, J. O. (1966), "The Determination of Long-Term Credit Standing with Financial Rations." *Empirical Research in Accounting/Journal of Accounting Research* 4(Suppl.):44–62.

Kaplan, R. S. and G. Urwitz (1979), "Statistical Models of Bond Ratings: A Methodological Inquiry." *Journal of Business* 52(2):231–261.

Lewin and Associates (1981), *Studies in the Comparative Performances of Investor Owned and Not-for-Profit Hospitals.* Washington, DC.

Long, H. W. (1976), "Valuation as a Criterion in Not-for-Profit Decision Making." *Health Care Management Review* 1(3):34–52.

Metz, M. (1983), "Trends in Sources of Capital in the Hospital Industry." In American Hospital Association, *Report of the Special Committee on Equity of Payment for Not-for-Profit and Investor-Owned Hospitals*, Appendix D. Chicago: AHA.

Morrisey, M. A. and J. A. Alexander (1985), "Hospital Entry Into Management Contracts." Working paper, University of Alabama at Birmingham, October.

Mullner, R., P. S. Levy, D. Matthews, and C. S. Byre (1981), "An Investigation of Institutional Characteristics Associated with Response Rates in Mail Surveys of Community Hospitals." *Public Health Reports* 96(March/April):128–133.

Pinches, G. and K. Mingo (1973), "A Multivariate Analysis of Industrial Bond Ratings." *Journal of Finance* 28(March):1–18.

Sloan, F. A. (1987), "Property Rights in the Hospital Industry." In H. E. Frech, III (ed.), *Health Care Policy* (forthcoming).

Sloan, F. A., J. Valvona, and R. Mullner (1986), "Identifying the Issues: A Statistical Profile." In F. A. Sloan, J. F. Blumstein, and J. M. Perrin (eds.), *Uncompensated Hospital Care: Rights and Responsibilities.* Baltimore: Johns Hopkins University Press, pp. 16–53.

Thompson, P. M. (1986), *High Yield Tax Exempt Hospital Bonds: Rewards, Risks, and Benchmarks.* New York: L. F. Rothschild, Unterberg, & Towbin, January 6.

Valvona, J. and F. A. Sloan (1985), "Hospital Profitability and Capital Structure: A Comparative Analysis." Working paper, Vanderbilt University, December.

West, R. R. (1970), "An Alternative Approach to Predicting Corporate Bond Ratings." *Journal of Accounting Research* 7(Spring):118–129.

COMMENTS ON DIVERSIFICATION OF HEALTH CARE SERVICES

Jon B. Christianson

The paper by Shortell and colleagues is ambitious in its scope and addresses a subject of current policy interest. As stated by the authors, the goal of the paper is "to develop and test a model of the factors associated with the growth in out-of-hospital services" provided by hospitals. The unit of observation is therefore the hospital. The authors are primarily interested in "diversification," which they define as "the provision of out-of-hospital services by hospitals or hospital systems. These usually involve the development of new services for new markets." The policy importance of the research derives from the apparent ongoing consolidation of the industry into multiunit systems and affiliations (the speed at which this is occurring is a matter of debate. Gabel and Ermann (1984), for example, present data suggesting a relatively slow rate of growth for hospital systems). In particular, there is concern that for-profit systems may provide a different number and mix of out-of-hospital services than other hospitals. Their out-of-hospital service mix may emphasize especially profitable services and ignore marginally profitable ones. Therefore, if for-profit systems increase in importance in the future, communities may find themselves with a dif-

Advances in Health Economics and Health Services Research, Vol. 7, pgs. 111–114.
Copyright © 1987 by JAI Press Inc.
All rights of reproduction in any form reserved.
ISBN: 0-89232-573-9

ferent mix of out-of-hospital services (provided by hospitals) available than if, for instance, nonprofit hospitals continue to dominate the hospital marketplace.

The authors define three measures of out-of-hospital services as dependent variables in their analysis: the overall number of services provided, the number of "unprofitable" services provided, and the percentage of services offered for which at least some charity care is provided. Each of these variables was hypothesized to be related to the same set of independent variables, with the direction of effects hypothesized to be the same in each case. The objective functions of hospitals are not stated formally in the paper, so these relationships are not derived from any explicit maximizing theory of hospital behavior. However, particularly as they pertain to number of services, the independent variables included in the analysis and the direction of the hypothesized effects seem reasonable.

The authors utilize the number of out-of-hospital services as their overall measure of hospital diversification. This measure has a history of use in the industrial organization literature [see, for example, Scherer (1980)] as a proxy for firm diversification. However, it does have some limitations in interpretation since it essentially treats all out-of-hospital services offered by a hospital as equally important. For example, a hospital offering an ambulatory surgical center and an outpatient radiology laboratory is treated as "diversified" to the same degree as one offering a geriatric day care center and a sports medicine program. Yet the diversification activities of the first hospital are clearly more closely tied to a hospital's traditional mission and probably are more important and closely linked to the hospital from a revenue-generating perspective. This suggests two areas where the diversification analysis could be extended.

First, it would be useful to know whether specific mixes of out-of-hospital services were more frequently observed than others. Also, which services or service mixes have traditionally been offered out-of-hospital and which are relatively new areas of hospital endeavor? Does the model predict better for "traditional" or "nontraditional" out-of-hospital services? What are the dynamics of the diversification process? Since the questionnaire administered to hospitals by the authors provides the year in which the service was first offered, it would seem that the dynamic aspects of diversification could be addressed. This would be consistent with the paper's stated objective to model factors associated with the *growth* of out-of-hospital services.

A second area of potential extension relates to an alternative measure of diversification and the importance of diversification to the overall activities of the hospital. As Scherer (1980) observes, "Merely counting product lines exaggerates in some respects the overall significance of diversification, since most firms' product volume distributions are highly skewed, with a few product lines accounting for the bulk of sales or employment while numerous other lines are relatively small" (p. 75). This limitation can be avoided to some extent by calculating specialization ratios (U.S. Bureau of Census, 1972) or their counterpart, "diversification ratios." A hospital's diversification ratio could be defined as the percentage of total hospital revenues derived from out-of-hospital services. The authors collect information on the number of patient encounters or procedures for each out-of-hospital service at every hospital in their questionnaire. Using approximate "shadow prices," revenue projections for out-of-hospital services could be attempted and a diversification index for each hospital constructed for use as an additional dependent variable.

To investigate the question of whether for-profit hospitals and/or systems are likely to provide fewer "unprofitable" services, the authors count the number of unprofitable out-of-hospital services provided, where *unprofitable* is defined as having operating revenues exceeding costs over some historical period. Hospital respondents are asked to identify such services through the questionnaire. Defining *unprofitable* in this way is certain to make economists uncomfortable, since overall hospital profits may be enhanced by services classified as unprofitable, if they generate additional inpatient admissions. The authors admit to this possibility in their discussion, terming such services as "loss leaders" and distinguishing them from other unprofitable services. This distinction, however, seems not to have carried over into the empirical analysis, where loss leaders and truly unprofitable services apparently are added together to form the dependent variable. The more appropriate and interesting variable for policy purposes would be the number of truly unprofitable services.

The third dependent variable used in the study is the percentage of out-of-hospital services offered for which at least some charity care is provided. While this is again an interesting variable for policy purposes, it may be the outcome of a different aspect of the hospital's decision making from the first two dependent variables. It is not clear why the same set of independent variables would be expected to affect this outcome in the same way as the previously discussed dependent variables. For example, the first "environmental characteristic" entered as an independent variable is "median income adjusted by the area wage index." The authors expect it to be positively associated with the volume of out-of-hospital services provided, presumably under the assumption that higher income levels in a community will translate into a greater demand for out-of-hospital services provided by hospitals. No similar justification is developed for a positive relationship between median income and percentage of services for which some charity care is provided. In fact, the effect may be in the opposite direction for charity care. In communities with relatively high incomes, there may be less occasion to provide care on a charity basis, and therefore fewer services overall for which charity care is provided.

The empirical analysis yields several results that, if confirmed in subsequent work, have important implications. For example, investor-owned system hospitals offer fewer unprofitable services than freestanding voluntary hospitals or voluntary system hospitals. With respect to the overall number of services, there are no differences between investor-owned system and voluntary system hospitals, but there are differences between investor-owned system hospitals and freestanding voluntary hospitals. Therefore, as the authors observe, it is necessary to distinguish specifically between ownership form and system involvement. This is an important finding and a caution for others engaged in similar research.

Finally, the general lack of significance for the "strategy" variables is worth noting. Strategy, by its very nature, is difficult to capture in quantitative terms. The disappointing performance of these variables may reflect a failure to accurately capture strategic decision-making processes in hospitals. The prospector/analyzer/defender/reactor typology, which was developed in an analysis of the cigarette industry, may not transfer well to the hospital industry. Or strategic considerations may have been relatively unimportant to hospitals at the time the study data were collected but will become increasingly important in the future. This is an area within the overall model that clearly needs further investigation using other data sets and classification systems.

REFERENCES

Ermann D., and J. Gabel (1984), "Multihospital Systems: Issues and Empirical Findings." *Health Affairs* 3(1):50–64.

Scherer, F. M. (1980), *Industrial Market Structure and Economic Performance* (2nd Ed.). Chicago: Rand McNally, pp. 74–80.

U.S. Bureau of the Census (1977), "General Report on Industrial Organization." In *1972 Enterprise Statistics*. Washington, DC: U.S. Government Printing Office, 1977.

COMMENTS ON RATIO ANALYSIS OF MERGED HOSPITALS

A. Woodward

The paper by Mullner and Andersen has two purposes: to describe selected characteristics of hospitals and to examine financial changes measured by ratio analysis. I will briefly discuss some of the limitations of ratio analysis and then suggest how ratio analysis opens up interesting avenues for further research.

Mullner and Andersen begin with a useful distinction between a merger and a consolidation, based on the definitions of Finkler and Horowitz.[1] A merger is the acquisition of one hospital by another, whereas a consolidation is a combination of two hospitals to form a new entity. This study concerns the mergers of 100 hospitals (55 being acquired and 45 acquiring) and the consolidation of 62 hospitals into 32 new hospital entities.

After describing locational, institutional, and environmental characteristics of these mergers and consolidations, Mullner and Andersen present financial ratio analyses of the combined hospitals. They concludes that "no clear financial gains or losses characterized merging or consolidating hospitals either before or after merger or consolidation." However, they speculated that five years before a combination and four years following might

Advances in Health Economics and Health Services Research, Vol. 7, pgs. 115–117.
Copyright © 1987 by JAI Press Inc.
All rights of reproduction in any form reserved.
ISBN: 0-89232-573-9

be too short a period of time to uncover significant financial changes in institutionally and environmentally similar hospitals.

There may be another reason to explain the lack of significant financial change in hospital mergers and consolidations. Ratio analysis is used to flag certain financial trends or differences which require further investigation. A ratio that remains similar after a hospital merges or consolidates is not an indicator that no material financial change has occurred. For example, the current ratio trend could remain largely unchanged even though there are changes in certain items which influence the current ratio, e.g., long-term debt and fixed assets, if the effects of these items are offsetting.

Ratio analysis may not be adequate to uncover differences in financial conditions among hospitals (even if the hospitals differ by institutional and environmental characteristics). A study of financial, cost, and productivity ratios recently done by Levitz and Brooke[2] showed fewer significant differences between institutionally opposite hospitals than we might expect.

Levitz and Brooke studied the differences in the financial performance, cost, and productivity of 94 hospitals in Iowa differentiated into system-affiliated or independent institutions. Their findings from the financial ratios showed that only the capital structure ratios and certain profitability ratios were significantly different between the two types of institutions. None of the activity and liquidity ratios was statistically different.

The study of Levitz and Brooke suggests in a way parallel to Mullner and Andersen's work that ratio analysis serves as point of departure for further research. The system-affiliated and independent hospital financial differences may not be found in ratios for the same reasons that differences are not found in the ratios in Mullner and Andersen's study. To find financial differences may require the application of complex statistical analysis. Levitz and Brooke advance this possibility in their statement that "matching and multivariate statistical methods in subsequent studies may provide an understanding of the impact of system affiliation, independent of other factors."[3] I look forward to future work Mullner and Andersen to uncover the extent of financial changes in merged and consolidated hospitals.

NOTES

1.   The definitions of Finkler and Horowitz cited by Mullner and Andersen is consistent with industrial organization definitions: a merger appears to correspond to a conglomerate merger in industrial organization terminology, and a consolidation appears to correspond to a horizontal merger. See F. M. Scherer, *Industrial Market Structure and Economic Performance*, 2nd ed. (Chicago: Rand McNally, 1980), pp. 123–124.

2. Gary Levitz and Paul Brooke, "Independent versus System-Affiliated Hospitals: A Comparative Analysis of Financial Performance, Cost, and Productivity." *Health Services Research* 20, No. 3 (August 1985): 315–339.

3. Ibid., p. 337.

PART II:

BEHAVIOR AND PERFORMANCE

MULTIHOSPITAL SYSTEMS AND ACCESS TO HEALTH CARE

Mark Schlesinger, Judith Bentkover,

David Blumenthal, William Custer,

Robert Musacchio, and Janet Willer

I. INTRODUCTION

The American health care system is in a state of flux. New financing and organizational arrangements are rapidly spreading, including systems of prepaid and prospective payment, self-insurance plans, and freestanding ambulatory care units. Many believe that these innovations portend major long-term changes in the American health care system, particularly affecting access to services. In a recent survey of health care providers and policymakers, 90% of the respondents suggested that access to care for uninsured and Medicaid patients would decline in the coming decade (Arthur Andersen & Co., 1984).

Perhaps the most pervasive institutional change in the past decade has been the growth of multifacility systems. Between the late 1960s and the mid-1980s, the proportion of short-term beds in system-affiliated hospitals grew from 5% to over 35%. Systemization has been most pronounced among proprietary facilities, the fastest-growing segment of the industry (Gray, 1983; Arthur Andersen & Co, 1984): roughly 80% of all for-profit short-term hospital beds are operated under chain auspices.

Advances in Health Economics and Health Services Research, Vol. 7, pgs. 121–140.
Copyright © 1987 by JAI Press Inc.
All rights of reproduction in any form reserved.
ISBN: 0-89232-573-9

How will this rapid growth of multifacility arrangements affect access to care? Past studies have pointed in conflicting directions, some suggesting that multifacility systems promote greater access, others indicating that system affiliation restricts access. No prior study has adequately controlled for the many other factors, aside from system affiliation, which may affect access to and utilization of services.

This paper is intended to develop a better understanding of the link between system affiliation by hospitals and access to care. More specifically, we will statistically estimate the relationships between hospitals' system membership, the probability that they are reported to discourage the admission of unprofitable patients, and the payor mix of physicians affiliated with those hospitals. Data for this study are based on reports from 3500 physicians in response to a 1984 survey conducted by the American Medical Association (AMA).

II. PAST RESEARCH ON SYSTEM AFFILIATION AND ACCESS TO CARE

A. Conceptual Issues

To provide access to unprofitable patients, a facility must be both willing and able to subsidize their treatment from the institution's surplus. Although there has been little analysis of the overall link between systemization and access, there has been considerable speculation about the impact of chain membership on both the size of the institution's surplus and its propensity to spend that surplus on unprofitable patients.

It is generally contended that multihospital system (MHS) hospitals will have larger surpluses from which to subsidize care. First, system affiliation is thought to allow the facility to capture economies of scale in the purchase of supplies and equipment (Brown, 1982; Vladeck, 1981), acquisition of capital (Cohodes and Kinkead, 1984), and, for smaller hospitals, in administrative overhead (Treat, 1976). Second, systems have the capacity to cross-subsidize individual hospitals, either from facilities operating in more profitable regions (Treat, 1976; Money et al., 1976) or through diversification into other services, including those outside health care (Ermann and Gabel, 1984; Coyne, 1982).

On the other hand, it is often argued that MHS hospitals will, for a given level of surplus, be less willing to spend funds subsidizing the care of unprofitable patients. This is thought to occur for a number of reasons. First, because system affiliation vests some control in the central office of the corporation, it is predicted to reduce the influence of the community in which the hospital is located (Ermann and Gabel, 1984; Starkweather, 1971). Under these conditions, the hospital may place a lower priority on care for the indigent (Kinzer, 1984). As Weinstein (1984, pp. 87–88) has noted:

> The MIOs [multi-institutional organizations] now seem to accept across the board the notion that the only health care they can provide in any significant way is that which returns them more revenue than their costs. Other care, whether needed or not, is relegated to some other provider or source... It is no longer indiscrete or inappropriate, from the provider's viewpoint, to refuse to offer care that is not being appropriately paid for.

Second, because larger organizations are generally more bureaucratically structured and hence bound by more formal rules and restrictions, physicians on the staffs of MHS hospitals are predicted to have less discretion over the types of patients which they are able to admit (Money et al., 1976). If these rules include means testing of patients prior to admission, they may restrict access. Finally, the large size of multihospital corporations is predicted to give them greater bargaining power in negotiations with state regulators (Ermann and Gabel, 1984; Vladeck, 1981). Moral suasion by regulators is increasingly seen as a means of encouraging providers to treat more unprofitable patients (Desonia and King, 1985). The enhanced bargaining position of MHS hospitals—leading to less regulatory pressure—may thus indirectly decrease the facility's willingness to treat the uninsured or underinsured.

A priori, then, one might expect to find that MHS hospitals were more able but less willing to subsidize access. The net effect of system affiliation would depend on the relative sizes of these two influences. This balance is likely to vary with market conditions (which may increase or decrease the hospital's surplus), the size of the subsidy required to encourage access, and other factors influencing the hospital's goals. For any given service, the net size and direction of influence of system membership must be determined empirically.

B. Past Empirical Studies

The influence of organizational structure on access to care has been measured empirically in three ways: (1) the propensity for facilities to locate in "unprofitable" areas; (2) the extent to which the facility offers services which are generally unprofitable; and (3) the willingness of the facility to admit and treat unprofitable patients (Schlesinger and Blumenthal, 1986). In each of these areas, there is a small body of evidence relating system affiliation to access to hospital services.

In their location decisions, MHS hospitals are particularly sensitive to financial incentives. On the basis of a voluminous review of literature on multihospital systems, for example, Ermann and Gabel concluded that:

Systems do not randomly choose where to locate, but self-select into favorable market areas. For example, for-profit systems tend to locate in fast-growing, less-regulated Sun Belt states and areas with lower Medicaid and indigent patient loads. (Ermann and Gabel, 1984, p. 59)

One empirical study has tested this proposition. The growth of for-profit chain hospital beds between 1972 and 1983 was regressed on a set of factors thought to foster that expansion, including prior entry by for-profit independent hospitals, the growth rate of population, the level of income, insurance coverage and Medicare spending, the average level of surplus in nonprofit hospitals, and the state's tax rate. For-profit chain hospitals were found to be more sensitive than their independent for-profit counterparts to both hospital profitability and average income in the state (Mullner and Hadley, 1984).

Another dimension of access involves hospitals' provision of services. One might expect that system-affiliated hospitals would offer the largest number of services, since economies of scale in access to capital have encouraged the expansion of new services (Cohodes and Kinkead, 1984). The provision of unprofitable services should therefore be the aspect of access most encouraged by system membership. Indeed, a number of studies indicate that MHS hospitals offer a wider array of services than do their independent counterparts (Sloan and Vraciu, 1983; Coyne, 1981; Bays, 1977).

None of these studies attempted to differentiate between profitable and unprofitable services. It is possible, however, to use data from one of these studies—Sloan and Vraciu's 1983 analysis of the hospital industry in Florida—to address this question. Past research indicates that a number of services are likely to be unprofitable for a hospital, because they are used disproportionately by uninsured or underinsured patients. These include inpatient dental care, emergency and outpatient departments, chemical dependency units, and emergency and outpatient psychiatric services (Sloan et al., 1986; U.S. Department of Health and Human Services, 1980; U.S. Department of Health, Education and Welfare, 1978; Rudov and Santangelo, 1979; Cannon and Locke, 1976). Focusing on these services, we find that there are pronounced differences in availability in system and independent investor-owned hospitals (Table 1), though both groups of hospitals were roughly equal in average size (Sloan and Vraciu, 1983). System membership thus appears to promote this aspect of access.

Another measure of the impact of system affiliation is captured by the proportion of unprofitable patients treated at the facility. Generally, this has been assessed by the proportion of self-pay patients and Medicaid recipients.[1] A number of studies have compared the payor mixes in for-profit MHS and nonprofit independent hospitals, and in general have found

Table 1.   For-Profit Hospitals with Services Used Disproportionately
by Indigents

Services Often Used by Indigents	Percent of Hospitals Offering Service	
	System Affiliated	Independent
Dental Care	40.0	15.6
Emergency Department	80.0	44.8
Outpatient Department	40.0	8.8
Chemical Dependency Unit	4.4	0.0
Emergency Psychiatric	15.6	0.0
Outpatient Psychiatric	6.7	0.0

Source: Calculated from Sloan and Vraciu (1983, p. 35).

few if any differences (Ermann and Gabel, 1984). These studies, however, confound differences due to ownership (for-profit vs. nonprofit) with those related to membership in a system. Since ownership has been shown to have demonstrable implications for access (Schlesinger and Blumenthal, 1986), it is essential to compare system and nonsystem hospitals of like ownership.

Some studies have made this latter comparison. The results for Medicaid enrollees have been mixed: some studies indicate the MHS hospitals serve a higher proportion of Medicaid patients (Sloan and Vraciu, 1983; Levitz and Brooke, 1985); others find the reverse to be true (Bays, 1977; Pattison and Katz, 1983). Since these studies examined hospitals in different states, it is unclear whether the differences in findings represent true differences in the propensity to serve less profitable patients or simply differences in the generosity of the Medicaid programs. These same studies found more consistent differences in treatment of the uninsured. All four studies found that chain hospitals treated an equal or smaller proportion of the uninsured than did independent hospitals of similar ownership (Table 2). These results also must be interpreted with some caution, however, since none of these studies controlled for differences in the extent to which uninsured patients might present themselves at the hospital or the market conditions (and hence the size of the hospital's surplus) under which the institutions were operating.[2]

In summary, there is some preliminary evidence—drawn from patterns of hospital location and treatment of uninsured patients—that system affiliation may make institutions more sensitive to financial incentives, and thus less willing to treat unprofitable patients. However, for at least some aspects of access, such as service availability, the lower costs of capital for MHS facilities may offset this enhanced sensitivity to financial concerns. Moreover, past studies in this area have some serious limitations. There have been very few studies of the effects of system affiliation on nonprofit

Table 2.   Proportion of Uninsured Patients in MHS and Independent
             Hospitals: Results from Past Studies

Authors of Study	Ownership of Hospitals	Decrease in Uninsured in MHS Hospitals	Measured in Terms of—
Bays (1977)	For-Profit	12%	Self-pay
Sloan and Vraciu (1983)	For-Profit	6%	Free care/ bad debt
Pattison and Katz (1983)	For-Profit	None	Charity care
Levitz and Brooke (1985)	Nonprofit[a]	47%*	Self-pay

[a]Some of the hospitals were managed by for-profit companies.
*Difference of means statistically significant at 5% confidence level.

hospitals. There have been no studies which have adequately controlled for factors other than system status which might affect the willingness or ability of the hospital to treat unprofitable patients. To provide a more accurate and more complete assessment of the influence of multihospital systems on access, we have estimated in this paper a set of regression models relating system status to several measures of access, as reported by the physicians affiliated with the hospital. These models statistically control for the influence of hospital attributes, the community in which it is located, and the regulatory and reimbursement systems under which it operates.

III.   PLAN OF ANALYSIS AND METHODOLOGY

A.   Measuring Access: Dependent Variables

Most past studies of access to inpatient care have used the hospital as the unit of analysis. Physician assessments, however, provide useful insights about access to hospital services. In this study, this aspect of access is measured by physicians' responses to the survey questions "Does the hospital (with which you are primarily affiliated) discourage admissions of Medicaid patients?" or "Does the hospital discourage admission of uninsured patients?" The hospital of primary affiliation was defined here as the hospital in which the physician reported spending the most time; doctors spent on average over 90% of their time in their primary hospital. As of 1984, 21% of responding physicians reported that their primary hospital discouraged admission of uninsured patients, while 6% reported restrictions on admission of Medicaid enrollees. We estimate below two regressions, one for the uninsured and one for Medicaid patients, relating system affiliation—as well as other characteristics of the hospital, physician, and the community in which they are located—to the probability that the responding physician reported restrictions on access.

There are important advantages in examining the perceptions of the physicians affiliated with those hospitals. First, in addition to formal institutional policies, physicians' admitting practices can also be affected by less formal administrative sanctions or moral suasion; these are not readily measured in surveys of hospital policies. Second, physicians have direct control over much of the admission and treatment process (Eisenberg, 1985). The effect of hospital policies on their behavior will thus largely determine the extent to which access has been restricted. Finally, restrictions on access will be experienced more by some types of physicians than others. Physicians with greater "bargaining power" (because of their seniority or the dependence of the hospital on them to admit a large number of patients) may be less likely to face constraints on their practices. Physician's reports of restricted admissions thus provide a useful measure of the extent to which access to care has been limited.

Physicians' perceptions of hospital access have some liabilities as well. Definitions of *discourage* may vary with social norms, and thus vary by region or the socioeconomic status of the community in which the hospital is located. In addition, perceptions are not always accurate. They may be influenced by the respondents' expectations of how the institution will behave. This is particularly likely if the hospital recently became affiliated with a system, and thus there is little "track record" on which to base an assessment of hospital policies.[3]

Hospital policies and practices may also indirectly affect access to physician services. Hospital services are complements to those offered by the physician (Pauly and Redisch, 1973). To the extent that doctors have difficulty admitting certain types of patients to the hospital, they will find it less attractive to treat those patients. Restrictions on hospital access are thus probably correlated with a reduced willingness by the medical staff to treat unprofitable patients. Hospitals may also attempt to affiliate primarily with physicians who treat few unprofitable patients.

To capture these indirect effects, we estimate below two additional regressions, having as dependent variables the proportion of the physician's practice that is uninsured or covered by Medicaid. In 1984, physicians reported on average that 10% of their patients were enrolled in Medicaid and 13% were uninsured. These payer mix variables were regressed against the system affiliation of the physician's primary hospital, again controlling for other characteristics of the hospital, the physician, the community, and reimbursement policies that may affect access to care.

B. Independent Variables: Influences on Access

1. System Affiliation. The hospital with which responding physicians reported a primary affiliation was categorized as being either a member of a multihospital system or an independent facility. Since, as noted previously, system membership may have an interactive effect with ownership, hospitals were grouped into six categories: independent nonprofit, independent public, independent for-profit, system nonprofit, system public and system for-profit.[4] The first of these was the omitted category in the regression.

2. Other Hospital Characteristics. The willingness and ability of hospitals to treat unprofitable patients depends on a variety of factors. Hospitals are assumed to be more willing to treat such patients if (a) they are highly dependent on low-income patients, measured here by a high proportion of Medicaid admissions; (b) they have few alternative sources of patient revenue, measured by the hospital's occupancy rate; and (c) there exist few alternative sources of care, measured by the proportion of hospitals in the county operated under public auspices.[5]

The larger the hospital's surplus, the more able it will be to subsidize care for unprofitable patients. Although we have no data on the size of this surplus, past studies indicate that this is a function of the facility's size, number of services, and teaching status (Sloan and Becker, 1984). In addition, the more competitive the market for hospital services, the smaller the surpluses are likely to be. The level of competition is measured here by two variables: the Herfindahl index for hospital admissions in the county[6] and the proportion of hospitals in the county operated under proprietary auspices. If investor-owned facilities, as has been argued, are more sensitive to market forces (Clarkson, 1972; Schlesinger and Blumenthal, 1986), it is possible that they create more effective competition and thus reduce institutional surpluses.

These hospital characteristics are included in both the hospital policy and physician payor mix regressions. Since, as noted previously, hospital services are complementary to physician services, factors which make the hospital less willing or able to treat unprofitable patients may well have indirect effects on physicians' willingness to serve those patients.

3. Community Characteristics. A variety of community characteristics are related to the number of uninsured patients who will seek treatment from hospitals or physicians. Proxies used here for the number of uninsured patients in the county are the average income of the county and the proportion of county residents who are black. In addition, because the poor may have readier geographic access to providers in urban areas, dummy variables are included for small (population under 1 million people) and large SMSAs (Standard Metropolitan Statistical Areas). The relative mix of uninsured vs. Medicaid patients is determined largely by the generosity of the state's Medicaid eligibility requirements (Granneman and Pauly, 1983). This is measured in our regression using two variables: the proportion of poor residents in the state who are eligible for Medicaid and the proportion of total hospital admissions in the county paid for by Medicaid.

Past studies also indicate that the willingness of physicians to treat Medicaid enrollees depends in part on the availability of more profitable patients and in part on the competitive pressures the physicians face (Sloan et al., 1978; Davidson et al., 1983). In the physician payor mix regressions these are measured respectively by the proportion of county residents over the age of 65 (a proxy for the availability of Medicare patients) and the number of physicians per 1000 county residents.

4. Reimbursement Systems. The willingness of providers to treat Medicaid patients is affected by the generosity of Medicaid reimbursment (Sloan 1983; Feder et al., 1984). Medicaid reimbursement may also affect, indirectly, willingness to treat the uninsured. Medicaid patients may act as either substitutes or complements for uninsured patients. If the first is the case, then the more generous the Medicaid reimbursement, the more providers spend time treating Medicaid enrollees and the less willing they are to treat the uninsured. If the latter is the case, higher Medicaid reimbursement produces a greater margin for providers, allowing them to cross-subsidize care of the uninsured.

In these regressions, "generosity" is measured in several dimensions. The generosity of payment to physicians is measured by the ratio of Medicaid to Medicare prevailing charges for a regular office visit. The generosity of hospital payment is captured by a dummy variable which is positive if the state uses prospective reimbursement or a limitation on inflationary increases for Medicaid hospital payments. Providers are less willing to treat Medicaid enrollees if the program involves restrictions or administrative requirements. To capture this effect, these regressions incorporate dummy variables representing requirements for prior authorization for procedures, outpatient surgery for selected diagnoses, or ceilings on the number of covered days of hospitalization.[7]

In addition, a number of other state reimbursement systems may affect access to care. These include all-payor systems for hospital reimbursement which pay for uncompensated care (New York, Massachusetts, Maryland, and New Jersey), a selective contracting system for hospitals serving Medicaid patients (California), insurance pools for "high-risk" individuals (seven states), and catastrophic insurance plans (Maine, Alaska, and Rhode Island). Dummy variables for each of these programs are included in the access regressions.

5. *Physician Characteristics.* As noted earlier, physicians with more status or more options for where they can treat patients may be less likely to face restrictions imposed by the hospital. Physicians with relatively few unprofitable patients in their practices may also be less likely to encounter restrictive policies. In these regressions, professional status is measured by length of time in practice. Options for treating patients are measured by the number of hospitals at which the physician has admitting privileges. The physician's payor mix is captured by the proportion of Medicaid or uninsured patients in their practice. In addition, physicians who are reimbursed in relation to the hospital's profitability may be less likely to encounter restrictions on admissions. A dummy variable is therefore included representing this method of compensation.

In addition to these variables, the physician payor mix regressions incorporate a number of other characteristics of responding doctors which past research has shown to be related to the propensity to treat Medicaid patients (Sloan et al., 1978; Davidson et al., 1983). These include the physician's specialty, sex, training, and employment status. Female physicians treat, on average, a higher proportion of unprofitable patients. Board-certified physicians generally see fewer of the less profitable patients, graduates of foreign medical schools more. Doctors employed by hospitals are thought to have less financial incentive to avoid unprofitable patients; those working in health maintenance organizations (HMOs) tend to treat fewer uninsured or Medicaid enrollees.

The willingness of physicians to treat Medicaid patients also has been shown to be a function of the economics of the physician's practice (Sloan et al., 1978). These same factors are likely to effect willingness to treat the uninsured. This is captured in these regressions by the availability of patients (measured by the waiting time for an appointment) and the costs of practice, proxied by the average wage rate of the physician's employees.

Finally, the propensity to treat unprofitable patients will likely be affected by hospital policies. As noted earlier, if the hospital discourages admissions for certain types of patients, they will prove more difficult for the physician to treat and thus, all else equal, less attractive. Similarly, if the hospital pays the physician through incentives related to hospital profitability, treating the uninsured may also seem less desirable. For these reasons, physicians' reports of these institutional policies are included as variables in the payor mix regressions.

C. *Description of Data and Statistical Techniques*

Data for this study are drawn from three sources: (1) the 1984 AMA Socioeconomic Monitoring System (SMS) Core Survey; (2) the 1982 AHA Annual Survey of Hospitals; and (3) the 1982 Area Resource File (ARF).

The SMS is a quarterly telephone survey program that collects information from a stratified random sample of nonfederal patient care physicians, excluding residents. The sample is stratified by specialty and census division. Data collected include information on physician training and demographic characteristics, income, practice expenses, visits, hours worked, payor mix, and fees (Henderson and White, 1983). In 1984, 4002 physicians were interviewed during the core survey. This survey involved a supplemental series of questions on physicians' relationships with hospitals—developed in collaboration with the staff of the Institute of Medicine—that included questions about attempts by hospitals to discourage admissions by particular types of patients. Only 1% of the survey respondents asked this question refused to reply.

In addition, the SMS also collected information on the physician's primary hospital, allowing a merging of data from the 1982 AHA survey (the most recent hospital survey available at the time the combined data set was constructed). Merging data provided information on hospital ownership and system status, organizational structure, utilization, and service availability (Mullner et al., 1983).

The third data set contains county-level data on the distribution of health manpower and facilities as well as the economic and sociodemographic characteristics of the population. This ARF data file, compiled by the Division of Health Professions Analysis, Bureau of Health Professions, is a secondary data source utilizing information from a number of public and private data bases. Information on characteristics of state Medicaid and other reimbursement programs was obtained from published sources (Granneman and Pauly, 1983; Sawyer et al., 1983; Desonia and King, 1985).

After merging data sets, information for the access analyses was available for approximately 3000 physicians. Because the data were drawn as a stratified random sample of physicians, it is not fully representative of the hospitals in the United States. More specifically, large urban hospitals are overrepresented in the sample. Nonetheless, because responding physicians were affiliated with over 2200 separate institutions (roughly 38% of all short-term general hospitals in the country), we believe that this data set fairly accurately captures the ongoing effects of system affiliation on the delivery of health services.

Because the dependent variables in the hospital access regressions are dichotomous, these regressions were estimated using a probit technique.

Table 3.   Predicted Impact of System and Policy Variables on
Probability Hospital Reported to Discourage Access

	Type of Payor	
	Medicaid Patient	*Uninsured Patient*
Average for All Respondents	5.7%	21.0%
Marginal Impact of—		
Hospital Ownership and Control[a]		
For-Profit Independent	+0.8	+7.0*
For-Profit System	+1.1*	+11.9*
Public Independent	−0.6*	−3.9*
Public System	−0.9*	−11.8*
Non₁ rofit System	−0.3	−1.8
State Policy Variables		
Medicaid Hospital Payment		
Other Than Cost-Based	+0.5*	+1.1
Medicaid Prior Authorization	+0.6*	+3.5*
All-Payers with Uncompensated		
Care Provisions	−0.6*	+3.5*
Preferred Provider (California)	−0.7*	+2.5*
Catastrophic Insurance	−2.5*	−7.5*
Mandatory Risk Pool	+1.5*	+3.2*

[a]Compared to independent private nonprofit hospitals.
*Coefficient statistically significant at 5% confidence level.

Physician payor mix regressions were estimated using ordinary least squares.[8]

IV.   RESULTS OF THE REGRESSION ANALYSES

A.   Hospital Access Regressions

Selected coefficients from the hospital access regressions are reported in Table 3.[9] As anticipated, there is a pronounced, and interesting, interaction between system affiliation and ownership. For investor-owned facilities, chain membership is associated with a substantial (roughly 40%) increase in the probability that physicians will report that the hospital discourages admissions of uninsured or Medicaid patients. In contrast, for both private nonprofit and public hospitals, system affiliation is associated with a reduced propensity to screen out unprofitable patients.[10] Other characteristics of the hospital and local hospital market also had significant influences on patient access. Physicians affiliated with for-profit hospitals, regardless of system status, were the most likely to report restricted access, physicians at public institutions the least likely.[11]

State policies also have had a significant impact on access to hospital services. The less generous is Medicaid reimbursement (in terms of either lower payments levels or a larger number of administrative restrictions), the greater the probability of reported restrictions on both Medicaid and uninsured patients. A number of innovative state reimbursement systems, including all-payors systems, preferred provider arrangements, and catastrophic coverage, appear to enhance access to Medicaid services. Curiously, however, only catastrophic coverage seems to promote access for the uninsured.[12] Risk pools are actually associated with greater reported screening by hospitals. This probably reflects the fact that states experiencing access problems were the most likely to adopt such programs but that the very limited participation in most of these programs has done little to actually encourage access (Bartlett, 1985).

B. *Physician Payor Mix Regressions*

In the same way that for-profit MHS hospitals are more likely to discourage access of unprofitable patients than are proprietary independent hospitals, but nonprofit MHS hospitals less likely to adopt such policies, so too the use of incentive payments for physicians seems to be linked to a combination of ownership and system status. For-profit system hospitals are about 30% more likely to pay physicians as a percentage of gross or net department revenues than are investor-owned independent facilities, but nonprofit chain hospitals are less likely to use such incentives.

As seen in Table 4, policies discouraging admissions and incentive payment arrangements each affects the proportion of Medicaid and uninsured patients treated by affiliated physicians.[13] Physicians' willingness to treat Medicaid patients appears to be more sensitive to hospital admission constraints, treatment of the uninsured to incentive payments.

Apart from these policies, the system status of the hospital seems be linked to few differences in the payor mix of affiliated physicians. Curiously, physicians on the staff of public MHS hospitals appear to treat more Medicaid enrollees, but fewer of the uninsured than their counterparts affiliated with independent public hospitals. Physicians associated with nonprofit system hospitals do treat somewhat fewer of the uninsured than do doctors at independent nonprofit hospitals. It cannot be determined here whether these differences are the result of a selection process by which particular types of physicians affiliate with certain hospitals or are the consequences of policies and incentives other than those measured by this study.

Some state policy variables also have a marked impact on access to physician services. The more generous the Medicaid payments to physicians, the higher the proportion of Medicaid patients in the physician's practice. (Interesting, however, we do not observe the same cross-subsi-

Table 4.   Predicted Impact of System and Policy Variables on Physician
Payer Mix

	Type of Payor	
	Medicaid Patient	Uninsured Patient
Average for All Respondents	9.6%	13.0%
Marginal Impact of—		
Hospital Ownership and Control[a]		
For-Profit Independent	−2.3	−6.9*
For-Profit System	−0.5	−1.9
Public Independent	−0.5	+1.8
Public System	+2.3*	−2.2
Nonprofit System	+0.4	−2.0*
Hospital Policies		
Discourage Medicaid Patients	−2.6*	+0.1
Discourage Uninsured Patients	+1.3*	−1.5
Incentive Reimbursement for MDs	+1.3	−5.5*
State Policy Variables		
Increase Medicaid MD Payments from 50% to 100% of Medicare	+2.5*	−1.2
All-Payers with Uncompensated Care Provisions	+1.1	+4.3*
Preferred Provider (California)	+1.6*	−1.6
Catastrophic Insurance	1.4	+9.1
Mandatory Risk Pool	−0.1	−2.5

[a] Compared to independent private nonprofit hospitals.
* Coefficient statistically significant at 10% confidence level.

dization effect in ambulatory care that were found in hospital access—the generosity of Medicaid reimbursement seems to have little effect on the proportion of uninsured patients in the physician's practice.) A number of policies designed to promote access to hospital care seem to also promote access to physician services. This effect is most pronounced in the use of all-payors systems with uncompensated care arrangements, which are associated with a higher proportion of both Medicaid and uninsured patients treated by physicians.

V.   DISCUSSION AND CONCLUSION

On the basis of these findings, it seems clear that the ongoing expansion of multihospital systems holds potentially important implications for access to health care services. System affiliation affects the propensity of hospitals to adopt policies which directly discourage access to inpatient services. Affiliation also influences, in a variety of ways, the availability of physician services. Hospital policies appear to have an indirect influence on the willingness of physicians to treat patients. There are also some differences in physician payor mix which are associated with system affiliation by the primary hospital, but which seem unrelated to either the policies or institutional structures examined in this study.

It is important to recognize the limitations of this study. Because it is based on physicians' perceptions, these findings may be biased by physicians' expectations that may differ from actual performance. The study evaluates only some dimensions of access to care.[14] To the extent that system affiliation has a significant influence on either the location of the hospital or its ability to adopt services, the net effects on access may be either more or less favorable than those reported here. Finally, we are unable to measure the impact of access restrictions on patient well-being. If alternative sources of care are readily available, restrictions on admissions may not always be undesirable from society's perspective: the economies and other advantages of specialization may actually promote social welfare.

Nonetheless, we believe that the findings reported here are important for both public policy and for our understanding of behavior of health care institutions. Certain policy implications are clear. Whatever the advantages to society of specialization of health care providers, restrictions on access will often prove detrimental to patients' health (Schiff et al., 1986; Relman, 1986). To the extent that the growth of multihospital systems leads to more restrictions, policymakers must be increasingly concerned about patient welfare. Moreover, the magnitude of the effects estimated here probably understate the future impact of systemization. In 1983, hospitals and other providers were just becoming sensitized to financial incentives that might lead them to restrict access (Weinstein, 1985). In the past several years, the perceived competitiveness of the market for health care services has increased, and it is predicted to increase more in the near future (Arthur Andersen & Co., 1984). As competition increases, providers will become more likely to restrict access. The use of prospective payment is spreading from Medicaid to state and private providers. As shown here, prospective payment further encourages hospitals to discourage admission of both Medicaid and uninsured patients.

Policymakers can respond to these changes in a number of ways. Policies can be designed to make it financially more attractive to care for patients. Our findings suggest, however, that at least in their initial years, such programs have only mixed success at preventing further restrictions on access to care. Other policies can be directed more specifically at the type of institutional policies shown here to inhibit access. States could prohibit, or circumscribe, the ability of hospitals to deny access to care. States could make illegal various forms of incentive payment arrangements which seem to discourage physicians from treating uninsured patients. In fact, a number of states are considering, and a few have recently adopted, policies directed toward these ends.

Beyond these implications for policy, there are clearly questions requiring additional research. For example, it remains unclear why system affiliation is associated with fewer reported restrictions on admissions in private nonprofit hospitals but more in their for-profit counterparts. Undoubtedly this difference in policy stems from differences in the influence of the community or professionals on institutional behavior, but the exact nature of this relationship requires further study. In addition, it remains unclear whether observed differences in the behavior of physicians affiliated with system and nonsystem hospitals result from differences in who affiliates with a system hospital or differences in the incentives facing doctors once they join the medical staff. These are not questions which will be easily answered. The importance of these issues and their clear connection to system affiliation, though, makes these questions well worth additional investigation.

NOTES

1.   We recognize that not all uninsured or Medicaid patients are unprofitable to treat. Nonetheless, because Medicaid often pays at sharply discounted rates (Granneman and Pauly, 1983; Sloan and Becker, 1984) and because many of the uninsured fail to pay for care at all (Sloan et al., 1986), on average these patients are more likely to prove unprofitable. These measures thus seem reasonable proxies for inadequately compensated care.

2.   Two studies, controlling for these factors using regression models, have examined the effect of system affiliation on the propensity of facilities to treat the *most* profitable patients. A nationwide study of hospitals found that patient care reimbursed by charge-based payors represented a higher proportion of patients treated in nonprofit MHS hospitals (compared to independent hospitals of the same ownership), but a lower proportion in for-profit chain facilities (Renn et al., 1985). These differences were statistically significant at a 5% confidence level. A nationwide study of nursing homes found that chain-affiliated homes had a higher proportion of private pay residents (the most profitable group), but this difference was not statistically significant (Birnbaum et al., 1981).

3.   The data used in this study are based on a survey of physicians. Roughly a quarter of the cases represented multiple physician responses for a single hospital. One might anticipate that if responses were based more on expectations than on actual performance, there would be less agreement in the responses of physicians affiliated with a given institution. In fact, the agreement rates for system (64.7%) and independent (65.1%) hospitals were virtually identical. There was a statistically significant difference in agreement rates between private nonprofit (66%), public (71%), and for-profit (46%) hospitals. It was anticipated, however, that physicians affiliated with for-profit institutions would be less often in agreement. Past studies have shown that investor-owned hospitals are less likely than their nonproprietary counterparts to adopt institution-wide rules, being more likely to tailor practices to individual staff members (Clarkson, 1972).

4.   Public facilities were designated as nonfederal short-term general hospitals. Physicians in federal hospitals were excluded from the AMA survey on which this study is based. Long-term care facilities were excluded to make the hospital sample more homogeneous.

5. Historically, private hospitals have "dumped" unprofitable patients on public facilities (Silver, 1974) and the number of patients so transferred appears to be growing in recent years (Schiff et al., 1986).

6. This index ranges from zero to one. The closer the index is to one, the more concentrated and, in theory, the less competitive is the market for hospital services. We would therefore predict that there would be a negative relationship between this index and the probability that a hospital adopts restrictive admissions policies.

7. Only the first of these variables is included in the physician payor mix regressions—we anticipated that all three would have similar effects on physicians but that prior authorization would represent the most significant of these influences.

8. Because a number of physicians treated no Medicaid or uninsured patients, these payor-mix-dependent variables were actually distributed as truncated normal variables. Reestimating these regressions using a tobit package, however, produced no significant changes in the regression coefficients or standard errors.

9. For reporting of the complete regression results, see Schlesinger et al. (1986).

10. For all three types of ownership, the differences between MHS and independent hospitals were statistically significant only for uninsured patients.

11. Similar findings were recently reported in a study of hospitals' propensity to deliver uncompensated care (Sloan et al., 1986).

12. The higher probability of hospitals limiting access for the uninsured in states with uncompensated care pools is particularly surprising. This may reflect a selection effect—states with the largest problems may have been the first to adopt these arrangements. The extent to which hospitals have taken advantage of uncompensated care provisions, however, may have been limited by the nature of these programs. In three of the four states (Massachusetts, New Jersey, and Maryland), the costs of uncompensated care are built into the hospitals' prices. This puts hospitals with a substantial amount of uncompensated care at a competitive disadvantage when competing for privately insured patients under preferred provider arrangments. Hospitals may therefore forgo treating the uninsured, even with indirect compensation available.

13. For a complete discussion of the regressions on physicians' treatment of the uninsured, see Blumenthal et al. (1986); for a presentation of the regressions for Medicaid enrollees, see Bentkover et al. (1986).

14. In their recent study of hospitals' provision of unprofitable outpatient services, Shortell and colleagues (1986) reported findings very similar to those found here: for-profit MHS hospitals were the least likely to offer such services; nonprofit MHS hospitals, the most likely among private facilities.

REFERENCES

Arthur Andersen & Co (1984), *Health Care in the 1990: Trends and Strategies.* Chicago: Arthur Andersen & Co.

Bartlett, Lawrence (1985), "State Level Policies and Programs." In *Access to Care for the Medically Indigent: A Resource Document for State and Local Officials.* Washington, DC: Academy for State and Local Government.

Bays, Carson (1977), "Case-Mix Differences Between Nonprofit and For-Profit Hospitals." *Inquiry* 14(2):17–21.

Bentkover, Judith, Mark Schlesinger, David Blumenthal and Janet Willer (1986), "The Impact of Public and Private Sector Changes on Physician Participation in State Medicaid Programs." *Health Care Financing Review* (forthcoming).

Birnbaum, Howard, A. James Lee, Christine Bishop and Gail Jensen (1981), *Public Pricing of Nursing Home Care.* Cambridge, MA: Abt Books.

Blumenthal, David, Mark Schlesinger, Judith Bentkover and Robert Musacchio, (1986), "Physician Uncompensated Care." Unpublished paper, Center for Health Policy and Management, Kennedy School of Government, Harvard University.

Brown, Montague (1982), "Multihospital Systems in the '80s: The New Shape of the Health Care Industry." *Hospitals* 56(14):71–74.

Cannon, M. and Locke, B. (1976), "Being Black is Detrimental to One Mental Health: Myth or Reality?" Paper presented at the W. E. B. Du Bois Conference on the Health of Black Populations, Atlanta, December.

Clarkson, Kenneth (1972), "Some Implications of Property Rights in Hospital Management." *Journal of Law and Economics* 15(3):363–384.

Cohodes, Donald and Brian Kinkead (1984), *Hospital Capital Formation in the 1980s*. Baltimore: Johns Hopkins University Press.

Coyne, Joseph (1982), "Hospital Performance in Multihospital Systems: A Comparative Study of System and Independent Hospitals." *Health Services Research* 17(4):303–339.

Davidson, Stephen, Janet Perloff, Phillip Kletke, Donald Schiff, and John Connelly (1983), "Full and Limited Medicaid Participation Among Pediatricians." *Pediatrics* 72(4):552–559.

Desonia, Randolph and Kathleen King (1985), *Programs of Assistance for the Medically Indigent*. Washington, DC: Intergovernmental Health Policy Project, George Washington University.

Eisenberg, John (1985), "Physician Utilization: The State of Research About Physicians' Practice Patterns." *Medical Care* 23(5):461–483.

Ermann, Dan and Jon Gabel (1984), "Multihospital Systems: Issues and Empirical Findings." *Health Affairs* 3(1):50–64.

Ermann, Dan and Jon Gabel (1985), "The Changing Face of American Health Care: Multihospital Systems, Emergency Centers and Surgery Centers." *Medical Care* 23(5):401–420.

Feder, Judith, Jack Hadley, and Ross Mullner (1984), "Falling Through the Cracks: Poverty, Insurance Coverage and Hospital Care for the Poor, 1980 and 1982." *Milbank Memorial Fund Quarterly* 62(4):544–566.

Gray, Bradford (1983), "An Introduction to the New Health Care for Profit." In Bradford Gray (ed.), *The New Health Care for Profit*. Washington DC: National Academy Press, pp. 1–16.

Granneman, Thomas and Mark Pauly (1983), *Controlling Medicaid Costs: Federalism, Competition and Choice*. Washington, DC: American Enterprise Institute.

Henderson, Sharon and Mary Lou White (1983), "Design and Methodology of the AMA Socioeconomic Monitoring System." In Roger Reynolds and Jonathan Abram (eds.), *Socioeconomic Characteristics of Medical Practice, 1983*. Chicago: American Medical Association, pp. 1–10.

Kinzer, David (1984), "Care of the Poor Revisited." *Inquiry* 21(1):5–16.

Levitz, Gary, and Paul Brooke (1985), "Independent versus System-Affiliated Hospitals: A Comparative Analysis of Financial Performance, Cost and Productivity." *Health Services Research* 20(3):315–339.

Money, William, David Gilfillan, and Robert Duncan (1976), "A Comparative Study of Multi-Unit Health Care Organizations." In Stephen Shortell and Montague Brown (eds.), *Organizational Research in Hospitals*, Chicago: Blue Cross Association, pp. 29–61.

Mullner, Ross and Jack Hadley (1984), "Interstate Variations in the Growth of Chain-Operated Proprietary Hospitals, 1973–1982." *Inquiry* 21(2):144–151.

Mullner, Ross, C. Brye and C. Killingsworth (1983), "An Inventory of U.S. Health Care Data Bases." *Review of Public Data Use* 11(1):85–188.

Nutter, Donald (1984), "Access to Care and the Evolution of Corporate, For-profit Medicine." *New England Journal of Medicine* 311(14):917–919.

Pattison, Ronald and Hallie Katz (1983), "Investor-Owned and Not-for-profit Hospitals: A Comparison Based on California Data." *New England Journal of Medicine* 309(5):347–353.

Pauly, Mark and Michael Redisch (1973), "The Not-for-Profit Hospital as a Physician's Cooperative" *American Economic Review* 63(1):87–100.

Relman, Arnold (1986), "Texas Eliminates Dumping: A Start Toward Equity in Hospital Care." *New England Journal of Medicine* 314(9):578–579.

Renn, Steven, Carl Schramm, J. Michael Watt, and Robert Derzon (1985), "The Effects of Ownership and System Affiliation on the Economic Performance of Hospitals" *Inquiry* 22(3):219–236.

Rudov, Melvin and Nancy Santangelo (1979), *Health Status of Minorities and Low-Income Groups*, DHEW Publication No. (HRA) 79–627. Washington DC: U.S. Government Printing Office.

Sawyer, D., M. Ruther, A. Pagan-Berlucchi, and D. Muse (1983), *The Medicare and Medicaid Data Book, 1983*, HCFA Publication No. 03156. Washington, DC: U.S. Government Printing Office.

Schiff Robert, David Ansell, James Schlosser, Ahamed Idris, Ann Morrison, and Steven Whitman (1986), "Transfers to a Public Hospital: A Prospective Study of 467 Patients." *New England Journal of Medicine* 314(9):552–557.

Schlesinger, Mark and David Blumenthal (1986), "Ownership and Access to Health Care: New Evidence and Policy Implications." *New England Journal of Medicine* 314 (forthcoming).

Schlesinger, Mark, Judith Bentkover, David Blumenthal, Robert Musacchio, and Janet Willer (1986), "The Privatization of Health Care and Access to Hospital Services: Profits, Competition and Multi-Hospital Corporations." *Milbank Memorial Fund Quarterly* (forthcoming).

Shortell, Stephen M., Ellen M. Morrison, Susan L. Hughes, Bernard S. Friedman, and Joan L. Vitek (1986), "Diversification of Health Care Services: The Effects of Ownership, Environment, and Strategy." Paper in this volume; see Part I.

Silver, Laurens (1974), "The Legal Accountability of Nonprofit Hospitals." In Clark Havighurst (ed.), *Regulating Health Facilities Construction*. Washington, DC: American Enterprise Institute, pp. 183–200.

Sloan, Frank (1983), "Rate Regulation as a Strategy for Hospital Cost Control: Evidence from the Last Decade." *Milbank Memorial Fund Quarterly* 61(3):195–221.

Sloan, Frank and Edmund Becker (1984), "Cross-Subsidies and Payment for Hospital Care." *Journal of Health Politics, Policy and Law* 8(4):660–685.

Sloan, Frank and Robert Vraciu (1983), "Investor-Owned and Not-for-profit Hospitals: Addressing Some Issues." *Health Affairs* 2(1):25–37.

Sloan, Frank, Janet Mitchell, and Jerry Cromwell (1978), "Physician Participation in State Medicaid Programs." *Journal of Human Resources* 13(Suppl.):211–245.

Sloan, Frank, James Valvona, and Ross Mullner (1986), "Identifying the Issues: A Statistical Profile." In Frank Sloan, James Blumstein, and James Perrin (eds.), *Uncompensated Hospital Care: Rights and Responsibilities*. Baltimore: Johns Hopkins University Press, pp. 16–53.

Starkweather, David (1971), "Health Facility Mergers: Some Conceptualizations." *Medical Care* 9(6):468–478.

Treat, T. (1976), "The Performance of Merging Hospitals." *Medical Care* 14(3):199–209.

U.S. Department of Health, Education and Welfare (1978), *Health, United States, 1977–78*, DHEW Publication No. (PHS) 78–1232. Washington, DC: U.S. Government Printing Office.

U.S. Department of Health and Human Services (1980), *Health, United States, 1980*, DHHS Publication No. (PHS) 81–1232. Washington, DC: U.S. Government Printing Office.

Vladeck, Bruce (1981), "Multihospital Systems and the Public Interest." In Gerald Bisbee (ed.), *Multihospital Systems: Policy Issues for the Future*. Chicago: Hospital Research and Education Trust, pp. 63–76.

Weinstein, Isadore (1984), "The Future of the MIO in a Price-Competitive, Price-Driven Market." *Topics in Health Care Financing* 11(2):84–92.

HOSPITAL REORGANIZATION:
EXAMINING THE EFFECTS ON MEDICAL EDUCATION

Catherine M. Russe and Gerard F. Anderson

I. INTRODUCTION

A major public policy concern surrounding the changing hospital financing and delivery system is the continuing provision of certain services. In the past, medical education, biomedical research, technology development, and care for the poor and uninsured were financed by cross-subsidizing the cost of these services with patient care revenues. However, recent changes in hospital payment policies by both public and private payors have limited the ability of hospitals to cross-subsidize these products.

As financial constraints intensify and operating margins are diminished, some hospitals are beginning to reexamine this historical mission. The concept of "no margin—no mission" was discussed frequently at the conference. Other hospitals are changing their organizational arrangements to cope with the changing economic environment (Brown, 1979). Freestanding not-for-profit hospitals are joining not-for-profit chains, and investor-owned chains are expanding through the acquisition of freestanding not-for-profit facilities.

Advances in Health Economics and Health Services Research, Vol. 7, pgs. 141–156.
Copyright © 1987 by JAI Press Inc.
All rights of reproduction in any form reserved.
ISBN: 0-89232-573-9

These changes in organizational form are especially important given that changes in payment policy threaten to limit funding for certain services and given the concerns about the lack of commitment of hospital chains to medical education, biomedical research, technology acquisition, and care for the poor and uninsured. Investor-owned chains especially have been criticized for their lack of commitment to these services (Pattison and Katz, 1983; Relman, 1980; Ruchlin, Pointer, and Cannedy, 1983).

Numerous researchers have examined how ownership status can influence the hospital's commitment to providing uncompensated care (Commonwealth Fund, 1985b; Feder, Hadley, and Mullner, 1984; Feder, Hadley, and Mullner, 1986; Kelly, 1985; Sloan, Valvona, and Mullner, 1984). Many of these studies have the difficulty of separating the effect of hospital location from explicit managerial decisions concerning how much uncompensated care the hospital will provide, since most investor-owned hospitals are located in relatively affluent areas with good insurance coverage. Much less has been written about hospital chains' involvement with medical education, biomedical research, or technology development.

Medical professions education programs represent a major financial commitment in many teaching hospitals. This commitment to education is easily identified through the presence and scope of programs. In addition, the commitment to education is not a function of location, as is often the case with uncompensated care, but is directly under the control of the hospital management and trustees.

In this paper, we will examine the impact that changes in a hospital's affiliation or ownership status may have on health professions education programs. More specifically, we will examine the characteristics of not-for-profit freestanding hospitals that become affiliated with not-for-profit multihospital chains during the period 1976 to 1984. We will perform a similar analysis for not-for-profit hospitals that joined an investor-owned chain. In both cases we will be particularly concerned with whether the existence of educational programs plays a major role in the decision process. In addition, we will examine whether a change in affiliation or ownership status has an effect on the institution's commitment to education after the hospital has affiliated or merged.

II. BACKGROUND AND FRAMEWORK

There is widespread concern that changes in the payment system for hospital care are jeopardizing some of the services traditionally provided by hospitals and especially teaching hospitals (Commonwealth Fund, 1985a). Increasing scrutiny over the use of patient care revenues to finance medical education, biomedical research, technology development, and care for the poor, has raised concerns about the continued production of these services

(Andersen, Schramm, Rapoza, Renn, and Pillari, 1985; Freedman, 1985; Relman, 1984a; Relman, 1984b; Whitcomb, 1984). Conventional wisdom about hospital chains is that they are growing quickly, have greater access to capital markets, do not include large tertiary-care hospitals with teaching and research programs, and provide proportionately less care for the poor and uninsured than freestanding hospitals. Relman suggests that the growth of what he called the "new medical industrial complex" is particularly worrisome because it may put the interest of the stockholder ahead of the public and exercise undue influence on national health policy (Relman, 1980).

There is still debate, however, over the actual effect that changes in organizational form have on hospital services and outputs. In an extensive review of popular and academic literature, Ermann and Gabel report that chain hospitals appear to have greater access to capital markets but that the other factors suggested as advantages to system affiliation or adverse effects of system affiliation were not demonstrated to be significantly different between freestanding and system-affiliated hospitals (Ermann and Gabel, 1984). For example, most studies show no discernible difference in quality of care between the freestanding and system-affiliated hospitals. In general, however, little conclusive empirical work has been done, and articles on both sides of this controversy, particularly with respect to the effect of chain affiliation on hospital outputs, have generally been produced in the absence of empirical data.

A. Motivations for Hospital Affiliation

The decision of a not-for-profit hospital to affiliate with a not-for-profit hospital chain is a function of several factors. It may be useful to view this decision process from two perspectives: (1) that of the nonprofit, freestanding hospital, and (2) that of the chain with which the hospital chooses to affiliate.

Smaller hospitals have an incentive to join a chain to take advantage of any benefits that may accrue from economies of scale (Bennet and Ahrendt, 1981; Lewin, Derzon, and Margulies, 1981; Pattison and Katz, 1983). This includes combining materials and supply ordering and sharing resources such as materials management, information systems, and management expertise to reduce costs.

A second motivating factor is access to capital. Some hospital chains offer expanded access to capital to their affiliates (Hernandez and Hourie, 1979; Yanish, 1981). As the hospital's access to capital declines, the incentive to affiliate would increase. However, there are no data available that allow us to determine the relative access to capital. A proxy, the level of capital expenditures, provides information about where a hospital is in its capital cycle and what its future capital needs are likely to be.

Market share is another factor that may contribute to the decision for a hospital to affiliate. A hospital's market share is an indicator of institutional viability. As market share declines, it is expected that the likelihood of affiliation will increase possibly as a strategy to bolster its referral network.

A hospital's competitive position vis-à-vis the other hospitals in its market area should influence its decision to join a chain. A hospital with high costs relative to other hospitals in the area may be at a competitive disadvantage. Consequently hospitals with high costs relative to other hospitals in the area may be more likely to seek chain affiliation.

A final factor may be the presence of an educational mission (Anderson et al., 1985). Training residents and interns requires a diversity of patients to ensure quality education. As the proportion of medical students, interns, and residents per occupied bed increases, there will be a point at which there are not enough patients to adequately train these students both in terms of volume and breadth of exposure to different illnesses.

The greater the commitment to teaching, the less likely the hospital would be to abandon its teaching mission. Affiliation with a chain of hospitals could provide the teaching hospital with alternative delivery sites for educating interns and residents as well as other other health professionals. Thus, as size of the educational programs increases, there may be a need to seek a greater referral base or to provide alternative settings for education because of a decline in volume or type of patients required to train health care professions, and these hospitals might seek an affiliation. Our proxy for educational mission is the total number of residency and allied health programs offered in that hospital. In a separate specification we used the ratio of interns and residents per bed as a proxy for education.

B. Motivations for Not-for-Profit Chain Affiliation

Nonprofit multihospital chains have their own set of incentives for affiliating with a freestanding nonprofit hospital, which are sometimes in opposition to the freestanding hospital's incentives. For instance, the chain, in evaluating potential affiliates, would be most likely to seek out hospitals with low costs relative to other hospitals in the area.

A not-for-profit chain may be more interested in a hospital if it is perceived to provide high-quality medical care and enjoys a good reputation in the community. While there is no universally accepted measure for quality of care, accreditation by the Joint Committee on Accreditation of Hospitals (JCAH) can be used as a surrogate for quality of care. Chains generally strive to increase their market share as well, but generally do not pursue growth for growth's sake (Alexander et al., 1985).

Another factor the chain may look for in a desirable affiliate is the availability of a broad scope of services (Anderson et al., 1985). If a hospital in the same market area as other hospitals in the chain offers services that are not available elsewhere, or there is only limited availability in the chain, that hospital may be attractive to the chain. Incorporating into the chain a hospital that adds to the services available creates a fuller service organization. Thus, as the number of services offered by the chain in aggregate grows, patients requiring specialized services may not have to go outside of the chain to receive care. We would expect to see that as the number of services increases, the desirability of affiliation by the chain also increases.

A final factor to be considered by the chain when choosing a new affiliate is location. Is the hospital located in a market area the chain already believes is desirable? This could be the result of better insurance coverage, higher incomes, favorable regulatory environment, or a variety of other factors. We would expect to see a greater likelihood of affiliation if the market area has been penetrated by chains.

In summary, hospital preferences for affiliating with chains are expressed in Eq. (1), and chain preferences for affiliating with hospitals are shown in Eq. (2). However, since we are primarily concerned with the overall affiliation decision, the total effect is shown as Eq. (3).

$$\text{Hosp Aff} = f(\text{SIZE, CAP, MKT, COMP, EDUC}) \tag{1}$$

$$\text{Chain Aff} = g(\text{COMP, QUAL, MKT, SERV, LOC}) \tag{2}$$

$$\text{Aff} = j(\text{SIZE, CAP, MKT, COMP, EDUC, QUAL, SERV, LOC}), \tag{3}$$

where SIZE = number of statistical beds;
CAP = hospital's capital expenditures;
MKT = hospital's market share;
COMP = hospital's competitive position;
EDUC = hospital's commitment to health professions education;
QUAL = quality of care;
SERV = scope of services available in the hospital;
LOC = hospital location.

C. Change in Ownership Status

As an alternative to joining a not-for-profit chain, freestanding hospitals have the option of joining an investor-owned chain. Hospitals may choose to become members of an investor-owned chain for many of the same reasons they choose to join a not-for-profit chain. We anticipate that hospitals with the following characteristics will choose to merge with investor-owned chains: smaller hospitals, hospitals with a poor competitive position, hospitals with difficulty acquiring capital, and those with little or no teaching.

The ratio of capital expenditures to total hospital operating expenditures can provide insight into the hospital's capital structure and future financial needs and is an indicator of financial viability. The lower the ratio, the greater the financial distress of the institution and therefore the greater the likelihood of changing ownership status. To the extent that the free-standing hospital is an educational institution, the hospital may be reluctant to sell to a proprietary chain, fearing that the chain would not support the education programs in the future. Thus we would expect to see that as the teaching commitment increases, the likelihood for sale would decrease. Finally, the smaller the hospital, the more difficult it may be to compete in the market area if there are large institutions or chains that enjoy greater economies of scale. Thus we would expect to see a greater likelihood of changing ownership status as the number of statistical beds decreased.

D. Acquisitions by Investor-Owned Chains

From the perspective of the investor-owned chain, we expect that the decision to acquire an independent nonprofit hospital includes many of the same factors that the not-for-profit chain used in deciding to execute an affiliation agreement. In addition to these factors, we expect that education has a negative effect on the decision calculus, since education programs are generally perceived to add to total facility costs. We also expect that a hospital's desirability by patients and physicians in the market affects the acquisition decision. Occupancy rate can be used as a proxy for the hospital's desirability.

We have expressed the hospital's decision to sell its assets to an investor-owned chain in Eq. (4), the chains' decision to purchase a freestanding not-for-profit hospital in Eq. (5), and the complete acquisition decision in Eq. (6).

$$\text{Hosp Sale} = f(\text{SIZE, COMP, CAP, EDUC}) \tag{4}$$

$$\text{Chain Purch} = g(\text{COMP, QUAL, MKT, SERV, LOC, EDUC, OCC}) \tag{5}$$

$$\text{Own} = h(\text{SIZE, COMP, CAP, EDUC, QUAL, MKT, SERV, LOC, OCC}), \tag{6}$$

where
SIZE = number of statistical beds;
COMP = hospital's competitive position;
CAP = hospital's capital expenditures;
EDUC = hospital's commitment to health profession education;
QUAL = quality of care;
MKT = hospital's market share;
SERV = scope of services available in the hospital;

LOC = hospital location;
OCC = hospital's occupancy rate.

E. Effect on Education

The second major question we examine is how a change in organizational form can affect clinical training programs. Continued commitment to training medical professions education will be determined by a number of factors such as the cost of the educational programs, the financial strength, prospects for the hospital's future financial viability, and the hospital's definition of its mission. We will compare hospitals that changed status with hospitals that did not change status to determine if there is any change in commitment to education over time.

III. DATA

We used data from the American Hospital Association (AHA) Annual Survey of Hospitals from 1976, 1980, and 1984. We excluded the following hospitals from our file: those located outside the United States, psychiatric and substance abuse institutions, and federal hospitals.

Data on the number of clinical education programs offered at each hospital for each year 1976, 1980, and 1984 were added to the file. These data were gathered using annual directories of the American Medical Association on Allied Health Programs and on Residency Training Programs. The number of training programs for each hospital was recorded.

To examine the affiliation decision, sample and control groups were created for two time periods, 1976–1980 and 1980–1984. Because of changing definitions in the AHA file, a hospital was considered affiliated during 1976 if it was controlled by the Catholic Church or was a member of the Federation of American Hospitals, while in 1980 it was affiliated if it was a division of another corporation that owns or operates more than one hospital. For 1984, a hospital was affiliated if it was owned, leased, or sponsored by another corporation and had a multihospital system identification number.

The sample consisted of all hospitals that were freestanding not-for-profit at the beginning of the time period but had shifted to chain-affiliated at the end of the period. Preliminary analysis did not suggest any hospital characteristics that automatically prevented system affiliation; therefore, a nationally random sample of hospitals that were not-for-profit freestanding at both the beginning and end of each time period was selected for the control group.

The data used to examine the effect on changes in ownership status were organized similarly. First, files were created of all hospitals whose status shifted from nonprofit freestanding to for-profit chains in two time periods, 1976–1980 and 1980–1984. Hospitals in both groups were examined, and it became apparent that there was a geographic concentration of this activity. Preliminary analysis revealed that six states had over half the hospitals whose ownership status had changed during the specified time periods. In addition, these hospitals tended to have fewer than 250 statistical beds. The control group was created using hospitals that met the following specifications: (1) they must be in one of the six states; (2) they must have fewer than or equal to 250 statistical beds; and (3) they must have been nonprofit freestanding at the beginning and at the end of the time periods.

Tables 1 and 2 present the means and standard deviations for the independent variables used in each regression for the sample and control groups separately in the two periods 1976–1980 and 1980–1984.

IV. RESULTS

A. Factors Predicting Behavior

Table 3 presents the parameter estimates and standard errors from the logistic regressions used to estimate Eqs. (3) and (6).

The first regression predicts the affiliation decision between 1976 and 1980 and found three factors statistically significant. As the hospitals became less competitive in their local area, the probability of affiliation increased, suggesting that hospitals were affiliating to improve their competitive position. Affiliations were more likely to occur as the number of services available in the hospital declined, suggesting that hospitals were affiliating to broaden the scope of services offered. As the market penetration of chain affiliated hospitals increased, the probability that a hospital will affiliate increased.

In the second regression, which predicts the decision to affiliate between 1980 and 1984, competitive position and teaching status influenced the decision process. Most important for the study, however, is that education emerged as part of the decision calculus. The greater the commitment to allied health professions education, the more likely was it that a hospital would affiliate, although the number of residency programs was not a statistically significant factor.

The third and fourth regression models, which predict the probability of joining an investor-owned chain, were not statistically significant (p ≤ .05). Only one variable, hospital size, proved to be significant in either equation.

The most important result for this paper, however, is that education, measured by the total number of allied health or residency programs in a hospital, generally did not prove to be an important variable in the decision

Table 1. Hospitals Changing Affiliation Status

Variable	Proxy	1976–1980		1980–1984	
		Mean	Standard Deviation	Mean	Standard Deviation
Sample Group					
CAP	Capital Expend./Total Expend.	6.2%	4.6	6.8%	3.5
OCC	Occupancy Rate	66.6%	16.9	72.1%	16.10
COMP	Hosp. Expend. per Adj. Adm. / Expend. per Adj. Adm. County	1.00	0.25	.99	0.23
SIZE	BED Size	184	203	240	194
QUAL	JCAH Accreditation	73.0%	44.0	81.0%	39.0
SERV	Services Available	42.7	10.3	44.6	10.5
EDUC	No. Allied Health Prgms	0.39	0.99	0.47	0.93
EDUC	No. Residency Prgms	1.05	3.07	1.01	2.52
MKT	Hosp. Beds/Hosp. Beds County	40.8%	38.2	39.7%	35
LOC	Chain-Affiliated Beds / Hosp. Beds in County	18.4%	20	10.1%	15
EDUC	Interns & Residents/Bed	.019	0.05	.017	0.05
N	Number of Hospitals	176		199	

(continued)

Table 1. (continued)

Variable	Proxy	1976–1980		1980–1984	
		Mean	*Standard Deviation*	*Mean*	*Standard Deviation*
Control Group					
CAP	Cap Expend./Total Expend.	6%	2.9	6.2%	3.8
OCC	Occupancy Rate	72.4%	13.65%	76.2%	13.19
COMP	Hosp. Expend. per Adj. Adm. / Expend per Adj. Adm. County	.95	0.18	1.09	0.66
SIZE	BED Size	236.0	171.6	218.0	195.0
QUAL	JCAH Accreditation	89.0%	31.9	86.0%	35.0
SERV	No. Services Avail	46.7	9.40	44.2	9.66
EDUC	No. Allied Health Prgms	.5	.87	.28	0.65
EDUC	No. Residency Prgms	1.5	4.03	1.24	3.55
MKT	Hosp. Beds/Hosp. Beds County	43.8%	37.0	37.5%	37.0
LOC	Chain-Affiliated Beds / Hosp. Beds in County	14.4%	17.0	8.0%	14.0
EDUC	Interns & Residents/Bed	0.034	0.94	.036	0.084
N	Number of Hospitals	88		100	

Table 2. Hospitals Changing from Nonprofit to For-Profit Status

Variable	Proxy	1976–1980		1980–1984	
		Mean	Standard Deviation	Mean	Standard Deviation
Sample Group					
CAP	Percent Capital Expend.	6%	4.0	6.2%	4.0
OCC	Occupancy Rate	61.5%	11.3	59.4%	16.1
COMP	Hosp. Expend. per Adj. Adm. Expend. per Adj. Adm. County	1.09	0.23	1.06	0.53
SIZE	BED Size	104	48.2	107	80.6
QUAL	JCAH Accreditation	79.0%	41.0	75.0%	43.0
SERV	No. Services Available	38	5.01	37	6.99
EDUC	No. Allied Health Prgms	0	0	0.02	0.14
EDUC	No. Residency Prgms	0	0	0.08	0.27
MKT	Hosp. Beds/Hosp. Beds County	46.0%	41.0	50.0%	41.0
LOC	Chain-Affiliated Beds Hosp. Beds in County	21.0%	29.0	16.0%	24.0
N	Number of Hospitals	24		53	

(continued)

Table 2. Hospitals Changing from Nonprofit to For-Profit Status

Variable	Proxy	1976–1980 Mean	1976–1980 Standard Deviation	1980–1984 Mean	1980–1984 Standard Deviation
Control Group					
CAP	Percent Capital Expend.	4.9%	3.0	6.5%	4.0
OCC	Occupancy Rate	61.0%	16.2	59.9%	17.2
COMP	Hosp. Expend. per Adj. Adm. / Expend. per Adj. Adm. County	1.00	0.31	1.01	0.38
SIZE	BED Size	99	65.8	85.4	57.8
QUAL	JCAH Accreditation	79.0%	41.0	61.0%	49.0
SERV	No. Services Available	39.0	6.75	37	7.07
EDUC	Allied Health Prgms	0.09	0.36	0.04	0.26
EDUC	Residency Prgms	0.06	0.44	0.12	0.70
MKT	Hosp. Beds/Hosp. Beds County	49.0%	41.0	47.0%	40.0
LOC	Chain-Affiliated Beds / Hosp. Beds in County	21.1%	24.0	13.0%	19.0
N	Number of Hospitals	135		183	

152

Table 3.   Factors Affecting the Decision to Affiliate or Change Ownership
Status

| Variable | Regression Equations[a,b] | | | |
	1	2	3	4
Intercept	1.47	1.86	−1.14	−0.51
	(1.10)	(0.98)	(2.06)	(1.24)
SIZE per 100 beds	−0.00	0.00	0.01	0.01**
	(0.00)	(0.00)	(0.01)	(0.00)
CAP	4.65	5.89	8.37	−2.10
	(4.03)	(3.93)	(6.36)	(4.70)
MKT	−0.58	0.38	−0.29	0.62
	(0.49)	(0.41)	(0.68)	(0.45)
COMP	2.58**	−0.64*	1.05	0.34
	(0.92)	(0.32)	(0.64)	(0.40)
QUAL	−0.83	−0.51	−0.26	0.67
	(0.44)	(0.40)	(0.62)	(0.41)
SERV	−0.07**	−0.03	−0.07	−0.05
	(0.03)	(0.02)	(0.05)	(0.03)
LOC	2.73**	1.16	−0.27	1.04
	(0.99)	(1.04)	(1.10)	(0.82)
OCC	—	—	0.00	−0.00
			(0.00)	(0.00)
Allied Health Programs	0.23	0.41*	—	−0.99
	(0.20)	(0.21)	—	(1.09)
Residency Programs	−0.03	−0.07	—	−0.33
	(0.05)	(0.06)	—	(0.49)
Chi-square	30.25**	17.06*	9.87	16.42
	9 d.f.	9 d.f.	10 d.f.	10 d.f.

* $p \leq .05$.
**$p \leq .01$.
[a]Standard errors appear in parentheses.
[b]Columns:

   1.   =   Hospitals shifting from independent to chain-affiliated status between 1976 and 1980.
   2.   =   Hospitals shifting from independent to chain-affiliated status between 1980 and 1984 using the
            number of allied health and residency programs as the measure of teaching commitment.
   3.   =   Hospitals shifting from nonprofit to for-profit status between 1980 and 1980.
   4.   =   Hospitals shifting from nonprofit to for-profit status between 1980 and 1984.

to affiliate with a chain or to join an investor-owned chain. Regressions
using the ratio of interns and residents per bed as the measure of education
were also estimated. In these models, education was also not an important
variable in the move to affiliate with or join a chain. In interpreting these
results, it should be remembered that the effect of omitted variables on
the included variables is dependent on the degree of correlation between

Table 4. Analysis of Variance of Changes in Education Program
Descriptive Statistics[a,b]

		1	2	3	4
F statistic		0.81	1.40	0.00	0.00
Mean	Control	.011	.05	.000	− 0.02
		(.928)	(.479)	(.244)	(0.33)
	Sample	.125	− .03	.000	− 0.02
		(1.263)	(.585)	(0.00)	(0.14)

[a]Standard deviations in parenthesis.
[b]Columns:

  1 = Change in education programs in hospitals that affiliated with a chain between, 1976 and 1980.
  2 = Change in education programs in hospitals that affiliated with a chain between 1980 and 1984.
  3 = Change in education programs in hospitals whose ownership status changed between 1976 and 1980.
  4 = Change in education programs in hospitals whose ownership status changed between 1980 and 1984.

the omitted and the included variables. Our expectation is that the addition of more variables would reduce the influence of education and not increase the effect (Anderson and Lave, 1986).

B. Impact on Educational Programs

To determine the effect that system affiliation and changes in ownership status have on the continuation of education programs, we did an analysis of variance on the change in the number of accredited allied health and residency programs available in the sample and control groups. In all four cases, comparing sample populations with control groups for hospitals affiliating and hospitals changing ownership status in both time periods, there was no significant change in the commitment to education. Of the hospitals that changed ownership between 1976 and 1980, none had residency or allied health programs. Similarly, there were very few hospitals in the 1980–1984 sample group with educational programs. Table 4 displays statistical values for this analysis.

V.   CONCLUSIONS

The results of our analysis indicate that education was not a major factor in the decision for hospitals to affiliate with a not-for-profit or an investor-owned chain during this period. In addition, educational programs were not affected by the change in organizational arrangements. This study examined a period when education was generally well funded during a period of cost-based reimbursement when there was no incentive for hospitals to diminish their commitment to education. However, financial incentives are changing. Funding for medical professions education programs by both the public and private sectors is diminishing and increasingly insecure. As hospitals with education programs face the possibility of decreased or nonexistent operating margins, a new mission may emerge. Because the future funding for education is still uncertain and because changes in hospital output may occur slowly, we would expect to see a lag in the change in educational programs for hospitals that have changed affiliation or ownership status. Consequently, this will be an area to watch in the event that hospital reorganizations continue and as methods of financing education change.

ACKNOWLEDGMENTS

The authors would like to thank Elizabeth P. Mann, Terry Mackey, and Nora Gruner for their strong support and assistance in the preparation of this manuscript.

The study was funded by the Bureau of Health Professions, U.S. Department of Health and Human Services, and the John A. Hartford Foundation.

REFERENCES

Alexander, Jeffrey A., Bonnie L. Lewis, and Michael A. Morrisey (1985), "Acquisition Strategies of Multihospital Systems." *Health Affairs* pp. 49–66.

Anderson, Gerard F., Carl J. Schramm, Catherine R. Rapoza, Steven C. Renn, and George D. Pillari (1985), "Investor-Owned Chains and Teaching Hospitals: The Implications of Acquisition." *New England Journal of Medicine 313*:201–204.

Anderson, Gerard F. and Judith R. Lave (1986), "Financing Graduate Medical Education." *Inquiry* 23(Summer):191–199.

Bennet, James and Karl M. Ahrendt (1981) "Achieving Economies of Scale through Shared Ancillary Services." *Topics in Health Care Financing 310*(3):25–34.

Brown, M. (1979), "An Overview." In S. Mason (ed.), *Multihospital Arrangements: Public Policy Implications*. Chicago: American Hospital Association.

The Commonwealth Fund (1985a), "The Future Financing of Teaching Hospitals." In *Prescription for Change*, Report of the Task Force on Academic Health Centers.

The Commonwealth Fund (1985b), "Health Care for the Poor and Uninsured." In *Prescription for Change*, Report of the Task Force on Academic Health Centers.

Ermann, Dan and Jan Gabel (1984), "Multihospital Systems: Issues and Empirical Findings." *Health Affairs* pp. 50–64.

Feder, Judith, Jack Hadley, and Ross Mullner (1980), "Falling Through the Cracks: Poverty, Insurance Coverage, and Hospitals' Care for the Poor, 1980 and 1982." In S. J. Rogers, A. M. Rousseau, and S. W. Nesbitt (eds.), *Hospitals and the Uninsured Poor: Measuring and Paying for Uncompensated Care*. New York: United Hospital Fund.

Feder, Judith, Jack Hadley, and Ross Mullner (1984), "Poor Hospitals: Implications for Public Policy." *Journal of Health Politics, Policy, and Law* 9(2):237–250.

Freedman, Steve A. (1985), "Megacorporate Health Care." *New England Journal of Medicine* 312:579–582.

Hernandez, M., and C. G. Hourie (1979), "Capital Financing by Multihospital Systems." In S. Mason (ed.), *Multihospital Arrangements: Public Policy Implications*. Chicago: American Hospital Association.

Kelly, J.V. (1985), "Provision of Charity Care by Urban Voluntary Hospitals." In S.J. Rogers, A.M. Rousseau, and S.W. Nesbitt (eds.), *Hospitals and the Uninsured Poor: Measuring and Paying for Uncompensated Care*. New York: United Hospital Fund, pp. 49–69.

Lewin, L., R. Derzon, and R. Margulies (1981), "Investor-Owned and Nonprofits Differ in Economic Performance." *Hospitals* pp. 52–58.

Pattison, Robert V. and Hallie M. Katz (1983), "Investor-Owned and Not-for-Profit Hospitals: A Comparison Based on California Data." *New England Journal of Medicine* 309(6):17.

Relman, Arnold S. (1980), "The New Medical–Industrial Complex." *New England Journal of Medicine* pp. 963–970.

Relman, Arnold S. (1984), "Are Teaching Hospitals Worth the Extra Cost?" *New England Journal of Medicine* 266:1256–1257.

Relman, Arnold S. (1984), "Who Will Pay for Medical Education in Our Teaching Hospitals?" *New England Journal* 226:20–23.

Ruchlin, H., D. Pointer, and L. Cannedy (1973), "Comparison of For-Profit Investor-Owned Chain and Non-Profit Hospitals." *Inquiry* pp. 13–14.

Sloan, Frank, Joseph Valvona, and Ross Mullner (1984), "Identifying the Issues: A Statistical Profile." Paper presented at Conference on Uncompensated Hospital Care: Defining Rights and Assigning Responsibilities, Vanderbilt University, April 6–7.

Whitcomb, Michael E. (1984), "The Federal Government and Graduate Medical Education." *New England Journal of Medicine* 311(20):1322–1324.

Yanish, D. Leigh (1981) "Pooled Assets Expand Debt Capacity." *Modern Healthcare* 11:86–88.

WALKING SOFTLY:

THE ROLE OF MANAGEMENT IN ALTERING PHYSICIAN PRACTICE PATTERNS IN THE HOSPITAL CORPORATION OF AMERICA

Diana Barrett and Paul H. Campbell

I. INTRODUCTION

The economic environment for all hospitals, whether nonprofit or proprietary, part of a multi-institutional system or autonomous, is rapidly changing. Successful hospital managers must respond to economic forces that seek to reduce inpatient acute care utilization, such as the new Medicare prospective payment system (PPS). Hospitals, in order to thrive, even survive, under new and very different economic incentives, arguably must have the cooperation of their medical staffs, who admit all patients for care and determine an estimated 60–70% of hospital costs through their ordering practices. Yet physicians, still by and large paid on a fee-for-service basis, face incentives that often conflict with hospital incentives. Furthermore, many fear the growth of economic partnerships between hospitals, especially investor-owned institutions, and physicians. Doctors and nonphysicians alike are concerned that access and clinical decisions will be adversely affected by the economic considerations of the firm (i.e., hospital, hospital system).

Advances in Health Economics and Health Services Research, Vol. 7, pgs. 157–178.
Copyright © 1987 by JAI Press Inc.
All rights of reproduction in any form reserved.
ISBN: 0-89232-573-9

Arnold Relman, writing in the *New England Journal of Medicine* (1980), issued the following warning: "That sentiment [for "commercial partnership"] may make for good working relations between hospital administration and medical staff, but it sounds precisely the wrong note for a private market in which the hospital is the seller, the physician is the purchasing agent for the patient and the public pays the major share of the bill."

Relman fears not only that economic linkages between doctors and hospitals may lead to the loss of clinical objectivity, (threatening the quality of and access to care), but also that the physician's public role as an impartial evaluator of "drugs, devices, diagnostic tests and therapeutic procedures" will be jeopardized.

While Relman (1980) deplores management intervention in clinical decision making in all hospital settings, he has voiced special concern about the nature and degree of that interaction in investor-owned chain operations like the Hospital Corporation of America (HCA). He has claimed that differences in ownership (i.e., not-for-profit vs. for-profit) have been associated with disparities in medical resource utilization even prior to the initiation of recent hospital cost-containment efforts such as PPS. His evidence includes that of studies by Lewin et al. (1981) and Pattison and Katz (1983), which found lower overall average length of stay and higher ancillary usage per day in investor-owned hospitals. Sherman and Chilingerian (1983), however, surveyed all of the often conflicting and flawed research on this subject and declared, "To date, there is no evidence that for-profits are immune from the power and independence of physicians. Hence, suggestions that ownership type and corporate controls can keep the physicians in check appear to be unfounded."

A current research project at the Harvard School of Public Health is employing case research methods to examine physician–hospital relations in HCA, the largest investor-owned hospital corporation in the world. This writing describes the economic challenges faced by HCA administrators and admitting physicians, the research methods adopted for this study, which was initiated in April 1984, and some preliminary observations from the initial corporate level investigations.

Utilization per hospital inpatient case, at least in terms of average length of stay, has declined sharply for Medicare and non-Medicare patients nationally, as well as for HCA. This study attempts to find out if such changes at HCA can be attributed to managerial actions which have directly or indirectly motivated changes in physician medical practice. Have HCA administrators instituted tough new utilization control measures which compel changes in medical practice, and/or have they altered their basic (political/economic) relationship with physicians in some way to tie the doctors' financial success tighter to the hospitals' economic performance? In addition to the answers to those questions, we seek to understand the relationship between those two levels of intervention. Can a hospital manager, for example, fold physicians, however gently, into the hospital cost-control structure without substantially recasting the traditional "arms-length" management–medical staff relationship?

The resulting description of methods HCA managers are using to alter medical resource utilization will permit us to begin addressing another question: What advantages and disadvantages does the HCA corporate structure, primarily through size, diversity, and investor-owned status, appear to provide in hospital–physician relations? In other words, does HCA's corporate structure make it easier or harder to affect physician behavior? Similar investigations in autonomous nonprofit and proprietary institutions, as well as not-for-profit systems, will be necessary to validate the hypotheses generated.

Following a substantial period of orientation and investigation at corporate offices, field work is continuing in two stages, at two different "matched pairs" of general acute care hospitals, with the matching designed to reduce differences in observed medical utilization trends produced by environmental influences. Within each pair, however, the two hospitals differ substantially in terms of the rate of decline in Medicare average length of stay. The task at each stage is to describe how individual managers tried to alter physician behavior and to assess their relative effectiveness in reducing Medicare length of stay. Tentative hypotheses regarding the relative effectiveness of various managerial mechanisms are being developed at the first pair of institutions. Those hypotheses will then be refined and tested through a second set of hospital case studies and a subsequent survey of HCA divisional managers.

II. THE ENVIRONMENT

A. The Era of Cost Containment

Hospitals are now leaving an economic era shaped by third-party retrospective cost-based reimbursement, a method of payment which helped to foster increasingly higher levels of health care costs.

A variety of cost-containment measures have been initiated by government and industry to stem further cost increases. Since this is a study of how hospital managers can effectively influence the behavior of physicians, it is important to distinguish among those third-party policies directed at the hospital and those aimed at patients and/or physicians.

For example, employers and insurers, including Medicare, have sought to directly alter patient behavior by increasing the beneficiary's price sensitivity. This has generally been accomplished through increased deductibles and coinsurance levels, as well as greater relative beneficiary contributions toward monthly premiums. Research has shown that high copayments effectively reduce the average consumer's use of ambulatory services and his rate of hospital admission, but not his level of expenditures once admitted to the hospital (Newhouse, 1981). Rising premium contributions encourage the selection of less costly plans, health maintenance organizations (HMOs) in particular. The number of HMOs has risen sharply, largely as a result.

The Medicare prospective payment program, however, places the direct financial incentives to reduce utilization upon the hospital. This research, which seeks to describe the way hospital managers in turn try to influence physician behavior, therefore focuses upon the impact of provider payment mechanisms such as the prospective payment system (PPS). Failure to recognize the effects of other types of utilization-constraining methods (such as those aimed directly at consumers and/or physicians) in the selection of sample hospitals could distort the results of this study. This project separates reductions in medical utilization due to third-party pressures on hospitals from other influences on utilization.

B. The Prospective Payment Program: Hospital Incentives

Amendments to the Social Security Act in 1983 (P.L. 98–21) mandated the end of cost-based reimbursement for inpatient hospital care furnished under the Medicare program, and the initiation of a prospective payment system based upon diagnosis-related groups (DRGs). The new process, as of this writing in a three-year transition period, presents a change of considerable magnitude for hospital providers which now rely on Medicare for over 40% of their revenue. Their challenge results from the ultimate objective of the new law, to reduce the heretofore rapid rise in Medicare expenditures for inpatient hospital care while concurrently maintaining an acceptable level of quality and access to care for beneficiaries.

The PPS attempts to achieve this objective by fundamentally restructuring the basic economic incentives facing hospitals. Hospitals are now rewarded for reducing both the routine and ancillary costs for any given stay. In addition, because the system is case-based and restricted to inpatient care, the PPS also offers incentives to increase the number of admissions, especially for more profitable DRGs, and to develop new sources of hospital revenue from activities not constricted by DRGs, especially outpatient services.

These latter two revenue-enhancing measures complement a hospital strategy which reduces inpatient utilization per case and are therefore investigated as additional outcome variables. Doctors order not only hospital discharges but also admissions and outpatient procedures.

C. Physician Incentives

The economic and professional incentives facing physicians may be compared with those that the PPS has now introduced to hospitals:

Reducing inpatient costs per admission. Physicians in private practice operate on the same fee-for-service basis that they have since the implementation of Medicare in 1966. For many physicians the fees they generate from services provided in the hospital are an important part of their total income, often increasing with longer and more service-intensive stays in the hospital. Other causes for resistance to cutting inpatient utilization include the perceived legal need to practice "defensive medicine" and professional norms which emphasize high technology but not necessarily least costly interventions. Paul Elwood (1983), with these "counterincentives" in mind, declared: "Persuading doctors to control utilization for the sake of the hospital calls on administrators to perform nothing less than a diplomatic miracle."

Increasing hospital admissions. Doctors may appear to face the same incentives to increase inpatient admissions as hospitals; their incomes, like hospitals', rise with a greater inpatient caseload. In fact, however, this can be an area of substantial hospital–physician conflict. Hospitals may seek to enhance admission volume by expanding their medical staffs, hence possibly threatening the market share and income of established physicians. Thus, it is important to reflect upon the incentives of individuals and subgroups (such as current vs. new doctors), as well as the aggregate population.

Increasing outpatient services. Physicians can also be expected to resist expansion which appears to directly threaten their private practices. Vertical integration into nursing homes and home health agencies, therefore, will probably not be resisted by most physicians. Hospital-owned ambulatory care services, however, have a long history of medical staff resistance.

D. Hospital–Physician Reconciliation

While the Health Care Financing Administration (HCFA) has apparently given high priority to the development of a prospective payment system for physicians (as well as for nursing home and home health providers), there are currently too many unresolved technical problems preventing its implementation in the near future. Also, other third-party payors, including many HMOs, continue to pay doctors on a fee-for-service

Figure 1. Possible economic linkages

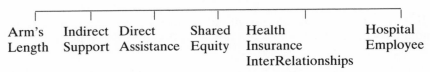

Arm's	Indirect	Direct	Shared	Health	Hospital
Length	Support	Assistance	Equity	Insurance	Employee
				InterRelationships	

basis. Thus the emerging economic environment of hospitals presents a major managerial challenge, i.e., the reconciliation of disparate incentives facing hospitals and physicians.

The literature offers innovations in organizational design toward this purpose, most all of which lead to the commercial partnership so feared by Relman (1980), from Elwood's MeSH plans (1983) and Shortell's Parallel Model (1985) to HMOs and preferred provider organizations (PPOs). Writers have also focused on ways to increase doctor cooperation within the traditional hospital design: Sandrick (1984), like Noie et al. (1983), argues for enhanced physician involvement in managerial decision making; Simendinger and Pasmore (1984) stress the manager's need for appropriate character traits and interpersonal skills; Egdahl et al. (1985) emphasize the need for enhanced information systems coupled with physician education; and Deal et al. (1983) promote the shaping, managing, and changing of institutional culture.

All the theoretical and empirical work in this area of hospital–medical staff relations was done before a full year passed under the new Medicare system. This research represents an initial effort to discover how well, in fact, these concepts work in the new economic environment. The investigation is proceeding at two levels, assessing recent changes in (a) the basic economic/political relationship between physicians and management in HCA hospitals; and (b) the operation of what has been termed "utilization review" (UR) and is now often called "utilization management."

The possible economic linkages fall along a continuum, from the traditional "arms-length" model on one end to hospital employment of physicians on the other (Figure 1). In between are various degrees of hospital indirect financial support (e.g., at-cost on-campus professional office space), to more direct assistance (e.g., no-interest loans and income guarantees), to shared-equity arrangements (e.g., joint venture construction/operation of diagnostic/treatment centers), and finally health insurance interrelationships (e.g., HMOs, PPOs). Politically, change might be evidenced in the way traditional "medical staff decisions" are made (e.g., admitting privileges) or in "management" decisions (e.g., nursing staff reductions). Of interest is the degree to which traditional and significant boundaries have been crossed in response to the new environment, with managers more involved in what have historically been viewed as medical issues, and vice versa.

Figure 2. Utilization management.

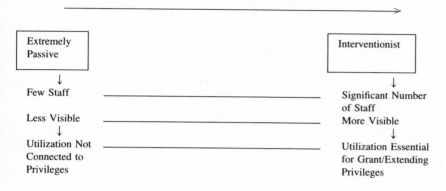

Utilization management (so-called since inappropriate utilization must be acted upon as well as "reviewed") also offers a spectrum for analysis, from extremely passive to highly interventionist (Figure 2). In the very passive model, hospital-employed review staff can be expected to be few in number and relatively less visible to physicians through personal or medical communication—in short, involved in a function relatively unchanged in design, processes, and capacity since the advent of the PPS. In a more interventionist model, very significant hospital resources, including staff, are expected for the tasks of identifying and resolving individual patient as well as physician and product (DRG) issues of unnecessary utilization. That relatively larger allocation of resources should be one of many indications of the great importance that senior management places on utilization management. The highly interventionist model would include doctors as far as legally possible in the hospital (i.e., management) control structure; questions of recruitment and continuing admitting privileges would be strongly influenced by the ability of the physician's practice to achieve hospital goals.

E. Current Trends in Hospital Utilization

Recent inpatient hospital utilization has shown some recent sharp declines, for the Medicare program, for patients under 65, and for the HCA, the focus of this study.

Since the inception of the PPS there has been a dramatic reduction in Medicare average length of inpatient hospital stay (ALOS). While the Medicare ALOS has been declining slowly since 1968, the rate of that reduction has markedly increased. Previous to 1984 the annual rate of reduction was 1.9%, according to HCFA figures; for 1984 the rate of decline jumped to 7.1%, as the ALOS fell to 8.8 days. More surprisingly (given the above mentioned economic incentives for both physicians and hospitals), admissions have also dropped off. The annual number of inpatient cases, which has generally grown slowly but steadily since the implementation of Medicare in 1966, declined 4% in all states in 1984, compared with a 2% growth during the previous year.

The American Hospital Association (AHA) has found an enhanced, but not nearly so dramatic, rate of decline in ALOS for the under-age-65 population as well. The ALOS, which had declined a total of 3.4% over the three year 1981–1983 period, fell 3.5% in 1984 alone. Admission rates for this group, which had also followed a long period of generally constant increase, leveled off during 1983 and began to decline through 1984.

Similar changes are found for HCA hospitals. The ALOS for all patients, which had changed very little from 1979 through 1982, fell nearly 2% in 1983 and nearly 7% in 1984. That fact, combined with lower admission rates, severely reduced hospital occupancy levels, which had already been below national averages. HCA hospital occupancy actually increased from 1979 to 1980 (2%), then dropped 1% in 1981, 5% in 1982, 4% in 1983, and nearly 14% in 1984. These declines have led to slowed earnings growth in 1985, the first slowdown since HCA was founded in 1968.

F. Institutional Strategy: The Hospital/Corporate Imperative

For hospitals the new economic incentives present large challenges. Consider the Medicare program; previously, declines in inpatient volume could be offset by proportionately greater costs per case. With the PPS fully implemented, however, the price per case is fixed and paid irrespective of the level of costs incurred. Overall losses for any institution will have to be covered by other sources at a time when private third-party payers are increasingly resistant to paying their own share, much less subsidies for others. Hospitals are concerned that private-payor subsidization of Medicare losses will make them less price-competitive for HMOs, the more recently developed PPOs, and direct hospital contracts with large employers, all of which control large blocks of patient volume.

Those hospitals and hospital systems able to increase outpatient services and their market share of inpatient admissions, while controlling utilization per case, should be able to generate profits which, if reinvested in "high-margin" services, promise to make the strong institutions even stronger. Their relatively solid financial position will make them much more likely to invest both in the plan and equipment required for technological/cosmetic renovation and the people resources required to offer increasingly sophisticated medical care. Those hospitals and hospital systems which cannot adapt face a relatively bleak future, one with continual trade-offs between economic survival and (a) quality of care standards and/or (b) access to care for the economically disadvantaged. Curtailment of services and eventual total shutdown and/or sale may result.

Both thriving and failing hospitals are to be expected in a structure designed to apply the rigors of the commercial marketplace. It is not yet clear which hospitals, or even types of hospitals, will thrive or fail. Nor has research revealed, from society's perspective, the effects of this economic rigor on the overall cost and quality of, and access to, the nation's medical care.

G. The Physician's Perspective

The hospital administrator's macro or institutional perspective has been contrasted with the physician's micro or patient-centered focus. Paul Starr (1982) has, in *The Social Transformation of American Medicine*, documented the increasing influence of M.D.'s in the health care arena over the last century. They have fought difficult social, economic, and political battles to maintain nearly total control over that "micro" doctor–patient relationship. Organizational intrusions, from the early industrial contract practices to modern HMOs, have been bitterly resisted. Physicians' general success in these struggles, Starr asserts, resulted from the general public's willingness to accept the expert–patient relationship they offered and their ability, within the profession, to act in concert. (The hospital's traditional and rather unique organizational design, which has provided physicians with the necessary support services without corresponding economic accountability, is evidence of that success.)

Why did they fight so hard and well? Certainly they appear to have been seeking far more than economic rents. Many physicians, including Relman, who was quoted earlier, believe that economic considerations do not have a place in clinical decision making; they perceive a "Berlin Wall" separating the micro and macro perspectives which should be maintained; (physician transgressors historically haven't been shot, but until recent court decisions they could lose medical society membership and hospital privileges).

They have a point. The members of Congress who voted for prospective payment believed that the health care market needed discipline, that there was substantial "fat" or "fluff" in the system which the new incentives could remove without touching the "core." Can that distinction be routinely made medically when there seems to be a very fine, often scientifically unproven line separating those services which truly enhance health status from those which do not? How would those same politicians perceive the need to separate the micro from the macro dimensions if they knew that medical decisions affecting their own morbidity or mortality were to be altered as a result?

H.   A Question of Accountability

The cost-containment mechanisms which this study focuses upon, those directed upon hospitals rather than patients or physicians, assign the accountability for medical practice quality to the hospital. Young and Saltman (1983) have clearly separated those cost elements which are primarily controlled by hospital managers from those controlled by the physicians, the environment, and third-party payors. They argue that a proper cost-containment methodology must align accountability with the ability to control costs. Managers, for example, should therefore only be held accountable for the price of inputs (labor, capital), while doctors should be answerable for the volume and types of services rendered. Because the PPS holds managers accountable for all three cost elements, Young and Saltman assert that it is doomed to failure; hospital administrators have never been able to significantly alter physician medical practices for the reasons described by Starr.

Starr (1982), however, at the close of his historical analysis, does argue that the social foundations of doctor's professional dominance have eroded over the past two decades; general public esteem has declined, and rapidly increasing numbers and types of physicians have rendered harmonious action very difficult. Meanwhile, it is very possible that the perceived importance of hospital administrators, in contrast, has been substantially enhanced by social pressure for cost containment. Does a major shift in the power balance between the two parties at least partially explain the radical and recent changes in hospital utilization (changes of course not evident when Young and Saltman wrote their articles)?

III. METHODS

A.   The Case Study Approach

Bonoma (1984) has found that case research is the investigator's tool of choice when the existing body of knowledge is insufficient to substantiate quantitative methods. Research into hospital–physician relations, especially within the context of dynamic environmental change, meets this criterion. We do not yet have the advantage of exploratory studies which identify and define the significant variables which could, for example, be assessed through survey research.

Hoaglin et al. (1982) cite the following quote from a publication of State Statistical Bureau of the People's Republic of China (1980) on the need for case studies as complements to statistical research:

The survey of typical cases is an important method to find out the circumstances and study the problems. Through the statistical tables, enormous phenomena may be understood but the causes of these phenomena and the problems behind them, and the means of solution cannot be found out simply from these date, and a detailed survey is indispensable. Therefore, besides making correct statistical tables, statisticians are asked to go deep into the realities of life and among the masses and conduct systematic and careful surveys of certain typical factories, shops and people's communes and acquaint themselves with the actual situation. For instance, where the statistical data of a certain area show an imbalanced fulfillment of the plan between the enterprises we would select three typical cases, the good, bad, and medium, reason why the good one is good and the bad one bad. In China there is a proverb: "The sparrow may be small but it has all the vital organs." After having dissected a few sparrows, one may have an idea about sparrows in general. With such rich and concrete materials, when combined with the figures from reporting tables, we can study problems, give the problems better explanations, and make suggestions on how these problems can be solved.

B. Corporate-Level Research

Information relating to corporation-wide operations was collected from the spring of 1984 through the fall of 1985 through the means of interviews, observation, and the review of secondary data. Multiple interviews were conducted with all key managers, including the current chairman of the board and chief executive officer (CEO), the presidents of the operating units (e.g., managed hospitals, owned hospitals, international operations), corporate vice-presidents responsible for critical functions such as development and finance, and a number of divisional (geographic) vice-presidents. The researchers also observed the proceedings at meetings of the board of directors, board committee sessions, and management conferences. Secondary data analyzed included financial and utilization information, annual reports, and corporate strategy statements.

Access to individuals and documents was assured by senior management of the company at the outset of this research and has not proven to be a problem despite the sensitive nature of the topic. The Harvard project is one of five university research endeavors initiated by HCA at approximately the same

While some data were collected on nearly all corporate activities, to enable the researchers to grasp the company as a whole the focus of investigations at both the corporate and hospitals has been the owned institutions (which have historically produced over 90% of the company's earnings). This has reduced the scope of research and therefore the generalizability of results. The managed hospitals, which now exceed their owned counterparts in number within HCA, are still directed at the policy level by their local nonprofit boards of directors, government entities, or private owners.

B.   Hospital-Level Research

1.   Sample Selection.   Our first challenge was the selection of sample hospitals. The need for similar economic environments limited us to a single state, which may also have implications for the generalizability of study results. Given our interests, we chose a state where we believe the environmental forces upon hospital utilization to be the greatest.

Once the state was chosen, quarterly data were collected on Medicare average length of stay for the period January 1, 1981, through December 31, 1985, for each HCA-owned hospital. Time series analysis was employed to measure the degree of change that has occurred since the new Medicare payment system was introduced in each hospital. We sought two matched pairs, as previously stated, which differed significantly in the degree of change in length of stay but were as similar as possible in other areas, such as bed size, teaching status, Medicare percentage of total patient revenues, Medicare average case weight, occupancy level, competition with other hospitals (within a 15-mile radius), HMO involvement, age of physical plant, HCA purchase date, and Medicare PPS implementation date.

Exhibits A and B display the Medicare average-length-of-stay data for the first pair of hospitals. Prospective payment was implemented in Hospital A, as noted, during the first quarter of 1984, and during the second quarter of the same year for Hospital B. Ordinary least squares regression found statistically significant (p < .01) changes in both level and slope were for Hospital A, but not for Hospital B. Checking for the significance of differences between the two hospitals, we drew 99% confidence intervals around the changes in level and slope found in Hospital A; the bounds thus computed did not contain the point estimates found for Hospital B. Thus, we were at least statistically certain that a difference exists between the two institutions. What time series analysis cannot reveal, of course, is the chain of causality behind such differences.

The two hospitals do not differ greatly in terms of bed size (both approximately 200 beds), teaching status, Medicare average case weight (a measure of relative resource consumption), occupancy levels, number of competing hospitals, HMO involvement, age of physical plant, HCA purchase date, or PPS implementation date. Probably the greatest difference found is Medicare as a percentage of totally patient revenue: 47% for Hospital A and 61% for Hospital B. One might assume that with a greater portion of revenues at stake, Hospital B might exert relatively greater pressure on its medical staff to reduce length of stay. That does not appear to be the case.

A number of factors must be considered when comparing hospitals' average lengths of stay. While the Medicare average case weights are

Exhibit A. Hospital A: Medicare average length of stay.

PPS INITIATED

INPATIENT DAYS

12 11 10 9 8 7

81 2Q 3Q 4Q 82 2Q 3Q 4Q 83 2Q 3Q 4Q 84 2Q 3Q 4Q 85 2Q 3Q 4Q

JANUARY 1, 1981–DECEMBER 31, 1985

169

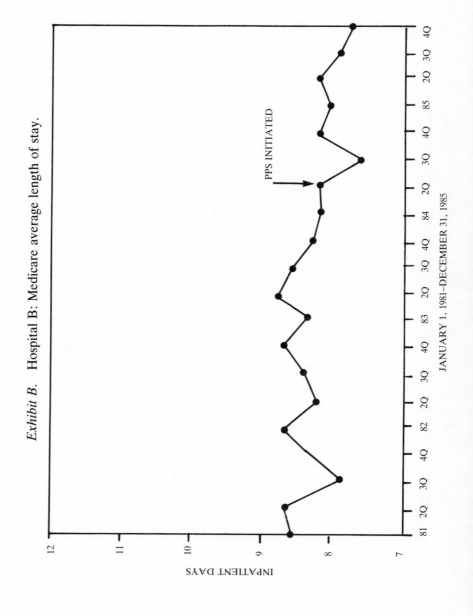

Exhibit B. Hospital B: Medicare average length of stay.

similar for the two institutions, one cannot assume that Hospital A was simply more generous in length of stay previous to prospective payment (case weights take into account resource demands other than length of stay and the two facilities may simply have different patient mixes), but that is a possibility. After all, it was in the hospital's financial interest, with the previous per diem cost-based retrospective payment system, to have longer lengths of stay, since greater costs are incurred by the facility at the points of admission and discharge. The possibility of relatively more unnecessary days prior to prospective payment therefore does not indicate any less willingness on the part of Hospital A's physicians to support the hospital's albeit changing strategy—quite the opposite. It may, however, indicate that Hospital B's medical staff may have fewer excess days to reduce in response to managerial or other pressure.

2. *Hospital Field Work.* Information is gained at the hospital level through interviews and secondary data analysis. Interviews to ascertain how hospital management is attempting to alter medical practice patterns include the administrator, chief of staff, assistant administrator, controller, director of nursing, director of social services, and utilization review (UR)– DRG coordinator. Secondary data of interest include financial and utilization reports and key committee minutes. The interviews and reports identify specific DRGs which have changed significantly the inception of the PPS. Physicians who have admitted substantial numbers of patients for those DRGs are then interviewed as well to determine just how their approaches to care have changed and to what causes they ascribe those alterations.

IV. PRELIMINARY OBSERVATIONS

While our hospital-level research has only begun, we can share a few preliminary observations regarding hospital–physician relations in HCA. Future investigation, in particular the interviews with attending physicians at the case study hospitals, will test and add depth to these first observations.

The company has traditionally sought to enhance its revenue base by recruiting physicians in needed specialties and by effectively building the institutional loyalties of the new recruits as well as established members of the medical staff. Below are comments which relate to that traditional strategy and its more recent embellishment; HCA now hopes the established "partnership" with its physicians will translate into a competitive advantage in hospital efforts to curtail utilization.

A. Physician Involvement in Managerial Decision Making

Writers cited above have advocated increased involvement of physicians in areas traditionally reserved for administration. Increased involvement, they maintain, leads to greater institutional loyalty and therefore reduced barriers when management attempts, for example, to increase outpatient surgery and reduce length of stay. The company has achieved this objective by altering the traditional formal governing structure of its owned hospitals as well as by undertaking informal means.

1. Formal Organization/Governance.

The literature on governing boards suggests that in general the traditional board of trustees in an autonomous institution has been a relatively risk-adverse decision-making body that usually does not have sufficient information to make important decisions. This leads to a power struggle between the medical staff and management. Decisions, when they are made, tend to be made in a slow and cumbersome manner. Physician representation is a relatively recent phenomenon and usually held to one or two members of the medical staff, when found at all.

The board structure at HCA is found at two levels: (a) the Corporate Board of Directors, concerned with overall policy, is far from hospital operations and primarily interested in financing and networking with other institutions; (b) the individual-owned hospital Board of Trustees has only advisory power and, along with the hospital Medical Executive Committee, commonly acts as the principal sounding board for management initiatives. This latter group is appointed by the hospital administrator and commonly consists of three or four members of the medical staff, an equal number of local business leaders, and the administrator himself. It is this body that usually makes the final decisions on medical matters—for example, the granting of hospital privileges (acting on recommendations initiated in the Credentials Committee and approved by the Medical Executive Committee).

One apparent difference found in comparing the traditional nonprofit hospital structure with that of HCA is the reduced decision-making involvement of community members other than physicians (and the businessmen mentioned above). Officials from local governments, related nonprofit institutions, and constituency groups, for example, are usually not included. Heavy medical involvement at the local level reflects the importance HCA places on doctors, who, as noted previously, largely determine the financial success or failure of each facility. Other community members—for example, officials from local governments, related nonprofit institutions, and constituency groups—are usually not included. One might hypothesize that this altered governing structure, which appears to limit input to medical and business interests, renders access for the medically indigent as far more vulnerable. Doctors have an obvious economic and professional stake in the real and perceived quality of the hospital in which they work; their financial stake in guaranteeing access to the economically disadvantaged is far less clear, in fact opposed.

The remoteness of the HCA Board of Directors means that hospital operational decisions which cannot be handled by the hospital administrator (e.g., financing a new ambulatory care wing) are made by a relatively few individuals with the relevant expertise in the Nashville corporate office. This tends to enhance at least the speed, if not also the quality, of decisions, factors which have taken on new value in the emerging competitive environment.

An interesting HCA innovation at the corporate level is the Board of Governors, established in the early 1970s and composed totally of physicians. This group does not appear to have a vital role in the operation of the corporation (its ostensible function is to address medical issues of importance to the company), but it does reinforce the significance that senior management places on the appearance of medical involvement at the highest level. So does the fact that two of the three founders of the company (the two who are still involved) are physicians. That fact is well known by doctors practicing at HCA hospitals; they are often quick to say that the company is "physician-founded."

2. Informal Organization. Often in HCA management meetings one hears a familiar adage: "The physician is our number-one customer." The administrator is responsible for putting this phrase into action throughout the hospital, through example and edict. Physicians with staff privileges in HCA hospitals rarely have trouble getting their input to administrators. The "open-door policy" applies to strategic issues as well as the much more common "parking space, operating room schedule" types of conflict. The inverse of this policy is also important: administrators are free to disagree with physicians and, if necessary, to alienate those whose interests do not appear to be congruent with those of the hospital. The corporate structure allows sufficient career mobility so that an administrator can move on after a short-lived but effective tour of duty.

There is no reason to ascribe the development of specific "core" corporate values, i.e., those that remain constant over time, to the investor-owned or multi-institutional form of a company like HCA. The constancy of any values, however, may well be facilitated by the corporate supervisory structure through mechanisms such as management meetings and hiring, transfer, and promotion policies. In HCA, where the decentralization of organizational responsibility and authority has been another guiding principle, attention to such values has always been important. Many important decisions (e.g., pricing strategy) are made at the hospital rather than at a regional or national level, according to a belief that better decisions are made closer to the action. Without a strong, centralized command center in the corporate headquarters dictating key policies for the individual hospitals, strong core values comprise the glue that holds the company together. A belief in the value of a single goal (budgeted earnings), rather than multiple performance measures which could dictate the means to that end, also results from decentralization.

B. Physician Recruitment

One approach to increasing both a hospital's inpatient market share and its outpatient activity is the recruitment of new medical staff members whose primary or specialty practices will accomplish both objectives. HCA hospitals have used financial incentives whenever necessary—e.g., low- or no-interest loans, free or low-cost office space, marketing assistance, part-time temporary employment in the emergency room, and guaranteed income levels, to cover some of the costs and many of the economic insecurities of the first year or two of practice. Autonomous nonprofit hospitals can and sometimes do offer a portion of the above enticements.

Another apparent advantage is the centralized physician placement network, one that doctors recognize through omnipresent advertisements in medical journals. Individual hospitals as well as nonprofit chains, however, can contract with private placement firms for the same service.

C. Ongoing Financial Ties

The financial relationship between the hospital and its admitting physicians may be characterized as either direct or indirect, depending upon whether dollars in fact change hands.

1. Indirect. Today, when hospital publications are filled with articles on joint ventures and MeSH options, it is sometimes forgotten that the economic prospects of hospitals and physicians have always been intertwined; the hospital is, after all, the doctor's workshop. What has changed is not the fact of interdependence but the level of environmental stress placed on that interdependence by disparate (hospital–physician) economic incentives. HCA has always well understood the importance of meeting physicians' needs; "get what the doctor wants" has been another guiding principle. High if not tops on the doctors' list is a modern, well-equipped facility within which to fully utilize his increasing technological skills. It is in this area that both HCA's investor-owned status and large size pay off in spades.

A company of over 400 hospitals (almost evenly split between owned and managed facilities), ambulance companies, regional reference labs, and assorted other enterprises can gain and retain expertise in finance, construction, and equipment purchase. After all, HCA has grown dramatically since 1968 by following a basic formula: selling stock, leveraging that equity, buying and building more and more hospitals, and passing on all the costs for both equity and debt financing to public and private payors. While the period of rapid hospital acquisitions and construction appears to be over, the ability to raise equity and debt financing is critical to the capital improvements necessary in the new environment. New and attractive outpatient surgery pavilions and on-campus medical offices are expensive. Economics of scale provide both access to larger amounts and more readily available capital and the kind of lower-cost/higher-quality construction that enhances bottom lines.

2. Direct. Underlying the management philosophy of strong decentralization (each hospital operates as a profit center) is another core value— that efficient productivity is maximized by releasing individuals' natural entrepreneural instincts. This tradition makes it all the easier to espouse what most doctors, and certainly organized medicine, want to hear—that HCA is 100% behind the continuation of fee-for-service medical practice. Only the minimum number of hospital-based specialists (e.g., pathologists) are employed directly by hospitals.

The predominance of fee-for-service is threatened in the wider world, however, on many fronts, from HMOs to hospital-owned ambulatory practices. HCA, however, has made very few moves in this direction beyond discussions and relatively recent ownership and management incursions into teaching hospitals.

Slightly less threatening to doctors (than HMOs and/or hospital-owned practices offering capitation/salary arrangements) are PPOs, which preserve the physician's fee-for-service model. They do, though, involve the hospital in the setting of doctors' fees (possibly with a discount) and certainly offer the structure (via utilization review) for future constraints on care. HCA, reading this as slightly less controversial, has developed PRIMED, a PPO first tried through company employees.

Another option to the direct employment of physicians consists of the myriad of joint ventures. The company's market research in this area finds that its own admitting physicians are significantly less opposed to the idea of joint ventures than to HCA ownership of medical practices. Joint ventures, perhaps with 80% HCA and 20% physician ownership, could for example, facilitate successful freestanding diagnostic and treatment centers. While a subsidiary, the Physicians Services Company, has been formed and discussions and experiments are pondered, HCA has not yet made major moves in this direction.

The contributions of HCA's size and structure in this area, therefore, relate to values and the ability to experiment in different environments. Economies of scale also enable the creation of an entity like the Physician Services Company, which can hire the relevant expertise should the corporation decide to make a major thrust.

D. Utilization Management

Our initial hospital research indicates that many (not all) HCA managers are indeed trying to affect physician behavior, to gain reductions in average len_th of stay. They are not getting results in this area by means of radically different systems; instead, they have added purpose to relatively old and previously ineffective utilization review (UR) and quality assurance (QA) systems. These systems offer at least the appearance of medical peer review, no matter how dominated they are by managers and nurses. In one 200-bed hospital, for example, there are six registered nurses, a medical record technician, and a secretary providing full-time "staff support" to the UR/QA efforts. Fully 100% of this hospital's cases are monitored on a concurrent basis. This is a radical increase in staffing and scope of review from the days when all impetus for review came from Professional Standards Review Organizations (PSROs) and the Joint Commission on Accreditation of Hospitals (JCAH). This beefed-up review system is then applied to physicians whose sensitivity to the cost-cutting importance of DRGs is reinforced in every professional journal.

Generalization from the above hospital to others in the HCA system, both as to the means and results of the "peer" review efforts, is a risky business, due to the realities of strong decentralization. In another hospital surveyed, for example, the review staff is approximately one-third the size of the first.

The company, however, has developed the tools with at least the promise of greater intervention. A computerized reporting system, initiated in all owned hospitals with the advent of the PPS, provides administrators with a great deal of data on individual admitting physicians—for example, the utilization of days and ancillary services as well as the costs, revenues, and profits per DRG. This system, however, has the weakness of relying on dubious Medicare cost reports (with a well-documented capacity to distort the true costs of services).

V. CONCLUSION

Why don't hospital administrators in general more aggressively control the ways their medical staffs practice? The answer is that doctors still operate from a very strong power base and they abhor any loss of what Starr called "professional sovereignty." They still determine admissions and outpatient service patterns. They can shift their share of inpatient practice from one hospital to another without notice and are increasingly capable of doing in their own offices what used to demand a hospital. In short, they can do a lot of damage.

The above comments, of course, apply to all hospitals with independent attending physicians. What is different about HCA is its size and investor-owned status, mentioned above as advantages. Veatch (1983) found that while organized medicine has been historically ambivalent regarding the profit motive for physicians, it has always been opposed to nonphysicians sharing in the income from physician labor as well as to nonphysician or "lay" intrusion into clinical decision making. HCA, with its large presence, attracts physicians' suspicions, which are in turn given voice by leaders like Relman.

Size also gives HCA a very large flank to defend. An initiative—for example, a joint venture with physicians in Georgia or the purchase of a medical practice in Alabama—might be very well accepted by the doctors in those immediate locales, but HCA has to be worried about how those stories will play before the national and very conservative audience.

Finally, those core company values promoting physician sensitivity and fee-for-service practice appear to keep a number of doors closed to HCA which are obviously open to others. Physicians' sensitivity is so high throughout the company that it is unlikely that major innovations in hospital–physician relations of the kind so feared by Relman will be pioneered at HCA. In fact, the company, at least for the foreseeable future, is likely to consistently lag behind the "hotdogs" in the not-for-profit group, those hospitals already "restructuring" and forming for-profit subsidiaries. HCA, seen as the threatening behemoth by many in the medical establishment, is likely to walk softly around both new financial linkages with doctors and "big stick" utilization management. As we begin our hospital-level research we are looking to test those predictions.

REFERENCES

Bonoma, Thomas (1984), "Case Research in Marketing: Opportunities, Problems and a Process Model." Unpublished paper, Graduate School of Business Administration, Harvard University, November.

Deal, T, A. Kennedy, and A. Spiegel (1983), "How to Create an Outstanding Hospital Culture." *Hospital Forum* (January/February).

Egdahl, Richard, et al. (1985), "The Cost-Effective Medicine Program." In R. Egdahl and Walsh (eds.), *Industry and Health Care*, Vol. 2. Cambridge, MA: Ballinger.

Elwood, Paul (1983), "When MDs Meet DRGs." *Hospitals* (December 16).

Feldstein, Martin (1971), *The Rising Cost of Hospital Care*. Washington, DC: Information Resources Press.

Freko, Deborah (1985), "Admissions Fall but Margins Are Up in '84." *Hospitals* (May 1).

Herzlinger, R., and J. Schwartz (1985), "How Companies Tackle Health Care Costs, Part I." *Harvard Business Review* (July/August).

Herzlinger, R. (1985), "How Companies Tackle Health Care Costs, Part II." *Harvard Business Review* (September/October).

Hoaglin, et al. (1982), *Data for Decisions: Information Strategies for Policymakers*. Cambridge, MA: Abt Books.

Levey, S., and D. Hesse (1985), "Bottom Line Health Care?" *The New England Journal of Medicine* (March 7).

Lewin, L., R. Derzon, and R. Margulies (1981), "Investor-Owned and Non-Profits Differ in Economic Performance." *Hospitals* (July 1).

Mitchell, Janet (1985), "Physician DRGs." *The New England Journal of Medicine* (September 12).

Newhouse J., et al. (1981), "Some Interim Results From a Controlled Trial of Cost-Sharing in Health Insurance." *The New England Journal of Medicine* (December 17).

Noie, N., S. Shortell, and M. Morrisey (1983), "A Survey of Hospital Medical Staffs. Part 1." *Hospitals* (December 1).

Pattison, R. and H. Katz (1983), "Investor-Owned and Not-For-Profit Hospitals: A Comparison Based on California Data." *The New England Journal of Medicine* (August 11).

Relman, Arnold (1980), "The New Medical Industrial Complex." *The New England Journal of Medicine* (October 23).

Sandrick, Karen (1984), "Medical Staff–Administration Relations Under PPS." *Hospitals* (April 16).

Scott, W. Richard (1982), "Managing Professional Work: Three Models of Control for Health Organizations." *Health Services Research* (Fall).

Sherman, H. and J. Chilingerian (1983), "A Look at the Myths and Half-Truths about Profit and Non-Profit Hospital Performance." Unpublished working paper No. 1511–83 Alfred P. Sloan School of Management, Massachusetts Institute of Technology (November).

Shortell, Stephen (1985), "The Medical Staff of the Future: Replanting the Garden." *Frontiers of Health Services Management* 1:3.

Shortell, S., T. Wickizer, and J. Wheeler (1984), *Hospital–Physician Joint Ventures*. Ann Arbor, MI: Health Administration Press.

Simendinger, E. and W. Pasmore (1984), "Developing Partnerships Between Physicians and Healthcare Executives." *Hospital and Health Services Administration* (November/December).

Starr, Paul (1982), *The Social Transformation of American Medicine*. New York: Basic Books.

Veatch, Robert (1983), "Ethical Dilemmas of For-Profit Enterprises in Health Care." In *The New Health Care for Profit*. Washington, DC: National Academy Press.

Wennberg, J., B. Barnes, and M. Zubkoff (1982), "Professional Uncertainty and the Problem of Supplier-Induced Demand." *Social Science and Medicine* Vol. 16.

Young, D. and R. Saltman (1983), "Prospective Reimbursement and the Hospital Power Equilibrium: A Matrix-Based Management Control System." *Inquiry* (Spring).

HORIZONTAL AND VERTICAL CONCENTRATIONS IN THE EVOLUTION OF HOSPITAL COMPETITION

David B. Starkweather and James M. Carman

I. INTRODUCTION

This paper reports on an investigation into the nature of competitive behavior among hospitals, in order to better understand and anticipate the effect of this competition on their efficiency and effectiveness. The study analyzed three communities chosen for their varying degrees of competitiveness in hospital and health care delivery. The research examined these communities with respect to (1) the environmental forces at work in the marketplace; (2) the changing structure of the hospital marketplace; and (3) the strategic responses of hospitals to their environments.

The study examined the nature of the three communities and their hospitals from 1979 to 1984. The conceptual approach was to assume that the market for hospital services was the appropriate one for analysis and then to investigate the efficiency of various competitive mechanism in allocating health care resources in the three markets. The focus was on where, when, and how market failures might develop. Failures include equity failures and dynamic efficiency failures as well as failures in allocative efficiency.

Advances in Health Economics and Health Services Research, Vol. 7, pgs. 179–194.
Copyright © 1987 by JAI Press Inc.
All rights of reproduction in any form reserved.
ISBN: 0-89232-573-9

The focus in this report will be on the role of both vertical and horizontal diversification and concentration among hospitals and on those aspects of these two phenomena that relate to environmental and market strategy, control of markets, and the positioning of hospitals relative to new and changing forms of health care financing and delivery.

The three study communities are all in California, since this state was among the earliest to develop a robust competitive environment in health care delivery.

Community A is a metropolitan city with a strong economy based on high-technology industry, a dramatic population growth, a high level of family income, and the presence of several large and progressive corporations each hiring more than 20,000 employees. Community A has 14 hospitals, of which 7 were examined. These included four not-for-profit hospitals (two community and two religious), two hospitals that were a part of a large health maintenance organization (HMO), and one government hospital providing care for the poor. This community was chosen for study because its hospital market was highly competitive at the outset of the period of time studied (see Table 1).

Community B is a smaller city serving a large agricultural area. It has a steady but undramatic population growth, a weaker economy, and an average family income of half that of Community A. There is no concentration of large employers in Community B because of its agricultural economy. All three hospitals in this community were examined. Community B was chosen because, for a portion of the time period studied, there was little competition among its three hospitals.

Community C is an isolated rural community with an agricultural economy and a stable population. There is a single hospital in the community. This community was chosen as a "control" community, since its single hospital appeared to hold a monopoly position and thus there was no competition.

II.   METHOD

The nature of competition was examined both within and between the three communities. For each community, information was collected from secondary sources on the financial performance of its hospitals and on the geographic origin of patients. These latter data permitted the calculation of market shares for the several hospitals and the determination of market concentration. The source of these secondary data was the California Health Facilities Commission. Primary data were obtained through interviews with hospital executives on the following dimension of competitive strategy: shifts in strategic direction, corporate reorganization, changes in management, involvement of the medical staff, investments in physical

Table 1. Summary Characteristics of Seven Hospitals in Community A, 1984

	Hospital						
	1	2	3	4	5	6	7
No. of Beds	204	403	329	352	305	338	208
Ownership	Church	Community	Church	Community	County	HMO	HMO
Occupancy Rate	75%	58%	75%	59%	79%	68%	71%
Special Strengths	Obstetrics Pediatrics Hemodialysis Rehabilitation Emergency service	Cardiac surgery Pediatrics Premature nursery Hemodialysis Psychiatry Obstetrics Alcohol chemical dependency Emergency service	Cardiac surgery Radiation therapy Hemodialysis Obstetrics Pediatrics Substance abuse Emergency service	Cardiac surgery Radiation therapy Obstetrics Psychiatry Pediatrics Hemodialysis Alcohol chemical dependency Emergency service	Tertiary burn Teaching Neonatal care Burn care Spinal cord treatment Occupational health Emergency service	Obstetrics Pediatrics Substance abuse Allergy Dermatology Ophthalmology Health education Emergency service	Obstetrics Hemodialysis Radioisotope therapy Psychiatry Cardiac catheterization Emergency service

181

plant and equipment, marketing research and promotion activities, horizontal mergers, vertical integrations or diversifications into nonacute services, geographic expansion, price contracting with large buyers of service, and involvement in the sponsorship of health plans.

All variables were classified and analyzed using the paradigm of environment, structure, behavior, and performance. For instance, numerous environmental factors influenced the rate of market entry from external and internal providers and allowed existing providers in growth areas to compensate for declining utilization rates with increasing primary demand. Changes in regulation and changes in Medicare and Medicaid programs were considered environmental factors.

Examples of structural factors are those that influenced physician loyalty to hospitals, which in turn led to competitive behavior that was more intense in the high-growth community than in the low-growth ones. Another structural measure was that of economic concentration, using the Herfindahl–Hirschman Index. This index measures both the number and size of competitors relative to the market.

Both environmental and structural factors led to competitive behavior that was more intense in Community A than in Community B and more intense in Community B than in Community C. This competition came from existing hospitals in the communities, physicians in the communities, and from limited entry from the outside. Further, the rate of change in behavior from cooperation to competition was greater in A than in B—although both responded to the changing environment.

These behavioral changes had an impact on the performance of the delivery system in these communities. The changes in performance moved in opposite directions for paying and nonpaying customers. Competition increased the quality and range of service provided to paying customers but decreased the access of nonpaying patients to private hospitals.

III.   FINDINGS

A.   An Overview

This paper reports findings only on Community A, since in this market the unfolding of competition with respect to horizontal and vertical concentrations was most obvious. (In Community B the unfolding of competition took place later in the period of time studied; in Community C it was largely nonexistent.)

Competition flourished in Community A, while the form of it varied. This was for several reasons. One was the strong economy, creating ample purchasing power. Another was the rapidly expanding population, creating opportunities for growth and diversity. Another was the presence of several large employers who, during this period of time studied, became knowledgable and aggressive with respect to the purchase of health care and health care insurance. This resulted in market pressures not previously experienced by hospitals for new bundles of services, new locations of service, and reduced prices.

The seven hospitals studied in Community A were of roughly similar strength; no single hospital dominated the market. There were relatively low levels of loyalty by physicians to single hospitals, coupled with overlapping medical staff memberships on the part of most physicians. In this way doctors and patients could move with relative ease among several of the hospitals. Table 2 shows that five of the seven hospitals studied were in relatively good financial shape except for the government one. [Data were not available for Hospitals 6 and 7, owned by a large health maintenance organization (HMO), because these data were not reported to the California Health Facilities Commission.] However, during the period of time studied the debt ratios for the community hospitals rose dramatically. There were relatively low occupancies across all hospitals, accentuated by a clear drop toward the end of the period of time studied. Even so, the most successful hospital financially was the one with a low occupancy (Hospital 2). This suggests that in a competitive arena, hospitals do not have to be full in order to be financially successful; indeed, excess capacity seemed to play a small role in the strategic decision making of the several hospitals. Instead, these hospitals concentrated on tight control of variable costs, yielding greater efficiency and productivity despite excess capacity.

Table 3 shows that at the beginning of the time period studied there was marked variation among the hospitals in their care for the poor, as measured by percentages of bad debt, charity, and contractual allowances. Further, during the course of the time period studied, two of the four eleemosynary hospitals (2 and 4) abandoned their social missions of care for the poor in favor of private patient business.

B.   Evolution of the Market

Against this backdrop of broad changes there was a more detailed unfolding of hospital competition in Community A. This occurred in three identifiable phases. In each of these stages the role of both horizontal and vertical mergers and diversifications was prominent. These changes in relationships between hospitals were stimulated by the new environment of competition created by changing regulations of federal and state governments. In turn, these mergers and diversifications fashioned and structured the nature of the competitive market. Thus in Community A they were central phenomena.

Table 2.   Overall Financial Performance of Five Hospitals,
Community A

	Hospitals				
	1	2	3[a]	4	5
1979/80					
Occupancy (%)	84	69	78	73	67
Gross Revenue ($000)	36,376	49,813	49,487	50,582	60,336
Net Operating Income ($000)	2,156	4,405	4,749	2,346	(17,588)
Operating Margin (%)	08	10	11	05	(38)
Nonoperating Margin (%)	02	02	01	004	23
Long-Term Debt/Unrestricted					
Assets	.04	.28	.05	.27	0
Accts. Rec./Total Current Assets	.73	.82	.91	.83	1.03[b]
1981/82					
Occupancy (%)	64	58	86	61	77
Gross Revenue ($000)	40,043	60,769	59,455	61,564	94,004
Net Operating Income ($000)	(754)	2,498	0	701	(19,086)
Operating Margin (%)	(02)	04	0	01	(22)
Nonoperating Margin (%)	NA	NA	NA	NA	27
Long-Term Debt/Unrestricted					
Assets	.52	.21	.45	.20	0.00
Accts. Rec./Total Current Assets	.77	.79	.82	.88	.74
1983/84					
Occupancy (%)	75	58	75	57	79
Gross Revenue ($000)	58,606	79,088	96,902	74,259	130,007
Net Operating Income ($000)	450	7,636	5,011	1,298	(23,226)
Operating Margin (%)	01	11	07	02	(27)
Nonoperating Margin (%)	04	03	02	03	16
Long-Term Debt/Unrestricted					
Assets	.50	.15	.48	.49	0.00
Accts. Rec./Total Current Assets	.73	.88	.90	.69	.89

[a]Statistics are for main hospital only; they do not include those of a subsidiary hospital (32 bed).
[b]Hospital error in reporting.

Stage I: Individual Competitors.   The first stage in this evolution occurred during 1979 to 1981. In this phase each hospital saw itself as an *individual competitor* and viewed all other hospitals likewise. This view was most pronounced among the four fee-for-service hospitals. There was proliferation of services among facilities, to the point of extensive duplication.

Every hospital except Hospital 6 went through a corporate reorganization. The motivations for these reorganizations varied, but in the main they had three purposes: (1) to provide a corporate form outside the hospital to undertake vertical diversification into ambulatory care, since certificate-of-need laws might block such developments if undertaken directly by the hospital; (2) to avoid 501(c)3 tax status jeopardy for "unrelated"

Table 3. Hospitals' Care of Charity and Government Patients, Five Hospitals in Community A

	Hospital					*State Avg.*
	1	*2*	*3ᵃ*	*4*	*5*	
1979/80						
Bad Debts and Charity Deductions/Charges	.05	.02	.03	.03	.10	
Total Deductions and Allowances/Charges	.24	.09	.15	.14	.20	
Percent Gross Revenue from Medicare	28	26	39	36	21	
Percent Gross Revenue from Medicaid	32	02	09	22	31	
1981/82						
Bad Debts and Charity Deductions/Charges	.04	.03	.03	.03	.07	.03
Total Deductions and Allowances/Charges	.23	.10	.11	.17	.20	.18
Percent Gross Revenue from Medicare	31	28	43	34	21	40
Percent Gross Revenue from Medicaid	30	06	07	22	42	16
1983/84						
Bad Debts and Charity Deductions/Charges	.04	.03	.02	.06	.17	
Total Deductions and Allowances/Charges	.29	.10	.18	.21	.36	
Percent Gross Revenue from Medicare	34	28	46	40	14	
Percent Gross Revenue from Medicaid	29	02	08	06	36	

ᵃStatistics are for main hospital only; they do not include those of a subsidiary hospital.

lines of business that might make money; and (3) to alter the decision-making process, particularly in regard to the medical staffs, since these bodies could block certain moves by the hospitals into lines of business considered by physicians to be their own.

Table 2 indicates that each hospital made a sudden and heavy commitment to debt, in some cases beyond the point of financial tolerance. These commitments were made to support heavy capital expenditures, which in turn were dictated by market-oriented strategic planning studies aimed at improving competitive position.

There was strong buildup in the management capacities of the several hospitals in the areas of strategic planning and marketing. This is shown in Table 4. These were occasioned by a shift in the outlook of these hospitals toward a market orientation. This was evidenced by (1) a change in the definition of customers away from doctors and toward private paying patients and potential patients; (2) an emphasis on assessment of these end-user target markets and their profitability; (3) limited vertical expansion through development or acquisition of preacute and postacute facilities and services; and (4) heavy promotional efforts.

However, during this first phase of individual competition there were several elements of a "perfect" competitive market that were missing. These included (1) the absence of well-informed corporate and individual

Table 4.   Additions to Seven Hospital Managements, Community A,
1979–1981

Hospital 1:	Promotion; medical care quality; marketing.
Hospital 2:	Planning; marketing; marketing and promotion.
Hospital 3:	Marketing; market assessment; planning; customer relations.
Hospital 4:	Marketing; market research; planning; medical care utilization.
Hospital 5:	Finance; advertising.
Hospital 6:	Customer relations; marketing.
Hospital 7:	None.

buyers; (2) a preponderance of comprehensive health insurance for consumers; (3) continuation of cost-based reimbursement to hospitals; and (4)
a relatively small number of sellers. These factors in combination yielded
a market in which price was not operating. None of the hospitals focused
on prices. Further, and consequently, there was (5) lack of emphasis on
productive efficiency within the hospitals; the hospitals did not know or
care about their marginal costs, so they could not make the calculations
necessary to determine output levels at which prices might be set in relation
to these costs. Finally, (6) there was incomplete and unsystematic competitor analysis. For this reason the fee-for-service hospitals failed to properly assess the impact that prepaid health plans and employer efforts at
cost containment might have on the market. Also some hospitals failed to
anticipate the responses that their own physicians would make as a result
of increasing doctor supply and increasing competition. Thus the market
in Stage I was not perfectly competitive, as the findings on price behavior
and other elements make clear.

Instead it was close to the model of "large-group" monopolistic competition (Chamberlin, 1933). The features were (1) continuing regulation;
(2) some product differentiation, with each hospital holding at least temporary monopoly over its available services due to certificate-of-need laws;
(3) close substitution between hospital services; (4) clear market definition
as regards subgroupings of fee-for-service, HMO, and government hospitals; and (5) demand and cost functions that were roughly the same for
all the hospitals. (Medicare-reported costs were similar among fee-for-
service hospitals. Each hospital assumed that demand was price inelastic
but could be supplier-induced.) Also, (6) there were a sufficient number
of hospitals relative to the market for each hospital to assume that specific
actions taken by it might go unheeded by its rivals or would not lead to
retaliatory measures that could impede its actions.

Each competing hospital appeared to have made the (naive) assumption
that price and product characteristics of its competitor hospitals were fixed;

thus its major strategy was one of product differentiation. Product differentiation was usually undertaken along service lines, with major attempts made in advertising, image making, and "brand name" promotion. A variety of differentiations were attempted. Some hospitals catered to a market interested in inexpensive services of lower amenity (Hospitals 1, 6, and 7); some catered to a convenience-conscious market with new services (Hospital 3); and still others attempting to add stylish gimmicks in hopes that these would attract patients or doctors (Hospital 4). Market analyses undertaken by two of the hospitals indicate that there was consumer recognition of these traits; but it is not clear whether or how consumers actually acted on these perceptions.

Finally, an element of the theory of monopolistic competition is that there will tend to be excess capacity, as firms will not construct minimum-cost sizes of plants or operate plants at minimum-cost rates of output. Such was the case in Stage I; the findings are clear as to the lack of concern for productive efficiency on fixed as well as variable costs, the medical arms race that propelled the purchase of expensive equipment without regard for its efficient use, and the efforts to expand capacity despite suboptimal and declining occupancies.

So on at least two counts—prices and capacity—competition during Stage I was not performing as it should. But Stage I was not a stable or permanent circumstance.

Stage II: Consolidation and Market Control. The second phase of evolving competition started in Community A in 1982 and 1983. This can be called the *consolidation and market control* phase. Normally this shakeout phase would have begun after the excess capacity created during cost-based reimbursement regulation, coupled with increasing marketing expenditures, had eroded net returns of the hospitals. While these effects were beginning to take place they were hastened by the special circumstances in California, where payment to hospitals for Medicaid patients was shifted from one based on cost to one based on individually negotiated prices. And coincident with this change in Medicaid reimbursement, private insurers were authorized by a new state law to negotiate with hospitals for PPO (preferred provider organization)-type price discounts. In addition, at the federal level, Medicare shifted from cost-based reimbursement to the prospective diagnosis-related group system. Thus, pricing behavior could no longer be ignored by hospitals, even though they were ill equipped for this aspect of competition. Further, employers and insurance companies began organizing new prepaid health plans designed to compete with the established large HMO and to reduce hospital utilization.

Several hospitals soon realized the futility of their "individual competitor" strategies of Stage I, given their diseconomies of small size and the heavy costs of monopolistic competition. So the strategy of several hospitals shifted from one of independent competition to one of controlling the marketplace through affiliation and merger. The stage had been set for this by the numerous individual hospital corporate reorganizations that had occurred during Stage I. In quick sequences there was a hospital merger among three fee-for-service hospitals (2, 4, and 10) and the initiation of merger talks between two additional hospitals (1 and 3), one of which had already assumed control of a third hospital (9). And the large HMO that owned Hospitals 6 and 7 stepped up its conversion of Hospital 7 from a combination of HMO and fee-for-service patients to an HMO-dominated operation. Further, the government hospital established closer program-matic affiliation with a nearby medical school hospital. In short order there was a de facto or projected restructuring of the market from 14 independent hospitals (seven of which were part of this study) to four hospital systems: two fee-for-service systems embracing seven previously independent hos-pitals, two HMO hospitals that were steadily expanding, and the county–university combination.

How these concentrations came about is instructive. In 1984 there was a combination between Hospital 2 and Hospital 4. (Technically, the com-bination was a holding company–subsidiary arrangement rather than a consolidation or merger, since both prior existing hospitals continued as operating entities even though they were owned and supervised by the parent corporation.) The idea of a merger was initiated by Hospital 4, stemming from a set of relationships that it had formed in prior years with Hospital 10. The management of Hospital 4 had been used by Hospital 10 as a consultant to develop its plans and strategies for the future. One feature of the recommended strategy was for Hospital 10 to seek an affiliation with another hospital in Community A in order to support its construction of a new facility in the high-growth northern section of the metropolis.

There was some expectation that Hospital 10 would seek this affiliation with Hospital 4, since the two hospitals had come to know each other through the planning process and since an advantage of such a merger would be the effective use of a 20-acre plot immediately north of Com-munity A that Hospital 4 had purchased in 1981—ideal for Hospital 10's relocated facility. But instead, Hospital 10 issued an RFP to several other hospitals. Both Hospitals 2 and 4 responded, along with others from inside and outside the community. Hospital 2 was chosen for affiliation, and it took place. It is through this process that Hospital 4 came to view Hospital 2 as a potential merger partner.

This possibility emerged from a market analysis undertaken by Hospital 4. Its management had come to place major stress on a future scenario wherein the competitive advantage of hospitals would depend on their presence in a broad enough geographic area to support contracts with a variety of employers and insurance groups. Hospital 4 had analyzed the 12 health service planning areas of Community A and calculated that a market share of at least 20% in each of the 12 would be necessary in order to hold a competitive position in the future. It calculated that the combination of Hospitals 4, 2, and 10 would obtain this 20% share in 9 of the 12 planning areas. Further, the combined efforts of the three could develop stronger positions in all 12 submarkets than any of the three hospitals could obtain separately or that any other hospitals could obtain separately. In the view of Hospital 4 officials, this combination of market spread and depth, when coupled with the "insurance arm" of an HMO, would place it and the other two hospitals in a strong position in the future prepaid and capitated health care environment.

Hospital 2 saw itself as a strong institution at the time of the proposed merger. It saw Hospital 4 as "hungrier" for an affiliation due to its poor inner-city location, its older plant, its aging physicians, and its high proportion of government-sponsored patients. To Hospital 2's chief executive officer (CEO) there were four short-run advantages of this merger: (1) provide for improved contracting capacity through the networking of the three facilities and the physicians related thereto; (2) obtain economies of scale in administrative areas and efficiencies through elimination of duplicate patient services; (3) improve borrowing capacity; and (4) help Hospital 10 with its construction in the northern sector, which of course would inure to Hospital 2's benefit as well. For the longer term, Hospital 2's CEO saw the merger as essential to survival because of the necessity to create a "critical mass" in the market and an asset base sufficient to generate revenue and obtain capital.

Another horizontal integration, between Hospitals 1 and 3, did not take place during the time of this study but was calculated by all parties to occur soon. Hospital 3 let it be known that if it did not affiliate with Hospital 1 it would do so with someone else. Hospital 1's CEO stated the integration would "definitely take place; the only question is form."

Hospital 3 saw the integration benefiting its own "tertiary facility" by linking it to Hospital 1's "bread and butter" operation. In this way Hospital 3 would obtain a feeder network and additional volume for its specialized programs. Hospital 3 also saw the affiliation as providing an opportunity to joint venture on several projects, such as a new hospital in the northern sector and an ambulatory surgery facility. Finally, Hospital 3 saw Hospital 1 as a network partner in a new HMO involving about 10 hospitals.

For Hospital 1 the proposed integration was based on "mutual needs." These included "external joint ventures," obtaining greater financial strength, and using Hospital 3's talents—while at the same time allowing each hospital the strengthened resource capability to initiate its own projects.

In summary, the relationship between Hospitals 1 and 3 was typical of proposed mergers between more powerful and weaker entities: the hospital that sees itself as the stronger anticipates a takeover, while the hospital that sees itself as weaker seeks a looser affiliation that will preserve some of its autonomy (Starkweather, 1981).

Shortly after the period of time examined in this study, Hospitals 1 and 3 acted in concert to obtain a certificate of need to build a hospital in the northern sector of the metropolis, in a town immediately adjacent to that in which Hospitals 10, 4, and 2 planned construction.

During Stage II some of the hospitals realized that their competitor analysis needed to include consideration of physicians as possible market entrants. But there was a dilemma. The new competitive environment made close hospital–doctor relationships more crucial. Thus in most hospitals physicians had been incorporated into the hospitals' strategic decision-making processes. Yet as the hospitals moved away from inpatient activity and toward ambulatory care they invaded the traditional domains of their doctors. Thus, hospitals faced the dilemma of whether the physicians on their own medical staffs were partners in strategy and market development or competitors.

At two of the hospitals the process of physician involvement in planning continued, even though the CEOs acknowledged that doctors were not accustomed to business-type decision making nor to "entrepreneurial discretion." One CEO lamented, "pretty soon the whole world knows what we are doing." At another hospital a variety of joint ventures were proposed. Its CEO stated that these were "to keep our existing programs and services from being unbundled to death. We need joint ventures with doctors so they won't peel away services that the hospital should provide."

In two other hospitals some of the physicians who were participating in hospital strategy bolted and set up ambulatory surgery facilities before the hospitals could enter the market. At one of these hospitals the CEOs charged these doctors with "insider dealing"; the hospital constructed a competing ambulatory surgery immediately adjacent to the one owned by some of its doctors. There then transpired bitter competition between the hospital and its doctors, including a price war complete with predatory pricing practices by the hospital calculated to drive the doctors out of business.

In short, there was during Stage II the emergence of physicians as competitive threats to hospitals, with different treatments of this problem by different hospitals. Since these competitors came from within their organizations rather from without, the process of competitive strategy development had to be altered.

In the main, during Stage II price competition was still not an important element of the hospitals' marketing mix. Hospitals were still trying to set noncontract prices as high as possible in order to offset contractual allowances on government-sponsored patients, and they begrudgingly granted price allowances to the state and a few PPO and HMO plans.

Two fee-for-service hospitals in Community A took another tack. The decision of the state to contract with individual hospitals for Medicaid patients provided a specific opportunity to the community and religious hospitals to determine whether or not they would continue their social missions of caring for poor patients. Two hospitals, 2 and 4, simply decided not to negotiate a contract, thus altering their longstanding missions and abandoning care of persons who could not pay full prices. As a consequence, these patients were shifted to one of the two religious hospitals and the government hospital. These shifted to one of the two religious hospitals and the government hospital. These effects can be seen in Table 3.

Stage III.   Expansion and Channel Control.   The third phase of evolution of hospital competition took place in Community A during 1984 and continued into 1985 and beyond. It is the *geographic expansion* and *channel control* phase. As with Stage II, this was brought on by market forces accelerated by a continuation of regulatory changes.

The circumstances now were (1) continuing and dramatic decline in hospital use; (2) excess capacity; (3) quick ascendency of private contracting by insurance companies, resulting in upwards of 35 PPO contracts in several of the hospitals and the calculation that in a short time more than 75% of their business would be "wholesale"; (4) realization by hospitals that marginal price contracting with the state for Medicaid patients was a long-term reality; and (5) the dramatic increase in forms of hospital payment—Medicare DRGs and HMOs—that shifted financial risk to hospitals and doctors.

During this third stage, hospitals shifted and broadened their emphases to include productivity. The need for serious cost management and cost containment had become obvious. Economies had to be found. Utilization control by physicians was now seen as extremely important.

But the major change in strategy was to focus on geographic expansion. Now the goal was to expand the geographic base of services needed to capture HMO and PPO contracts with employers whose employees lived in locations more widespread than the historic markets of individual hospitals. Now it was necessary to provide services over a broad geographic area—services for present and future HMO patients wherever they might live.

During this time numerous joint ventures were developed between hospitals and physicians, both for the provision of services in new geographic areas and in order to provide a hospital–physician unit for contracting with insurance companies and large employers. These activities constituted a new wave of vertical integrations in order to control and provide broader scopes of service. For example, the merger of Hospitals 2, 4, and 10 soon yielded a subsidiary new-venture corporation "dedicated solely to the development of innovative health services delivered outside of the hospitals." The first venture was a regional kidney stone center, developed in joint venture with numerous physicians. The next was a network of six geographically dispersed primary care centers, developed in joint venture with a medical group practice that admitted most of its patients to Hospital 4.

The marketplace was now seen as a health plan business. Future competition would most likely be among health plans rather than between individual hospitals or hospital systems. This begged the question of who would control the health plans. Market power would come to whoever controlled access to the ultimate consumer. The hospitals in Community A calculated that there were several possibilities on the provider side: local hospitals, local hospitals in collaboration with doctors, or coalitions of local hospitals with distant corporations. On the purchaser side there were the indemnity and prepayment companies and the large employers.

Thus the hospitals and the physicians in Community A were gearing up for two struggles: who would serve the new purchasers that were expecting hospital–doctor risk sharing and who would control the health plans that were usurping the patient "gatekeeper" role from doctors and becoming the channelers of patients to hospitals and doctors.

So all of the hospital systems in Community A either purchased or started to develop HMOs and other insurance vehicles—still another aspect of vertical integration and diversification.

By the end of Stage III the form of the hospital market had moved to one approximating a differentiated oligopoly. There was a small number of dominant firms. A substantial proportion of the total market was now being produced by four corporations. There was interdependence among the corporations, since each corporation was now forming its strategies with an eye to its effect on rivals, while also recognizing that its changes would elicit changes on the others' parts. Some economies of scale had been achieved. There were barriers to entering the market, notably certificate-of-need regulations and the heavy requirement on potential entrants to duplicate expensive facilities. Limit pricing did not appear as a tactic used by the oligopolists to bar entry. There was downward pressure on prices, stemming from the efforts of organized purchasers. But in general, pricing was not used by hospitals as a competitive weapon. Instead they used the less risky strategies of advertising and variation in service characteristics. They hoped to increase demand for their services at the same prices. And they hoped to induce users of hospital care to stick with their "brand name" even though many of the services among the several hospitals were essentially the same.

We would expect the profits of oligopolists to be higher on the average than they would be under perfect competition. We note from Table 2 that profits improved dramatically during Stage III. Of course, several things could have explained this result.

An interesting aspect of the oligopoly model is the degree to which there is price leadership among the firms and whether or not there is price collusion. One form of oligopoly behavior occurs when one dominant firm set prices for the industry. In neither Community A nor B was there a single, enduring price-setting hospital. Rather it appears that a barometer-firm situation existed where one hospital—not necessarily the largest nor most powerful—took the lead in making price changes that the others then considered following (Burik, 1983).

Price competition could have entered Community B in 1983, but it was voided. The state Medicaid program had previously been reimbursing hospitals on a percentage of each institution's full costs. It then shifted to a negotiated price arrangement where hospitals were encouraged to submit competitively priced bids for the state's business. However, the three hospitals separately decided not to enter the competition, based on certain information they had obtained from the local Health Systems Agency. This left the state no choice but to continue paying each on the basis of costs—which reimbursement was undoubtedly above what each would have obtained under some form of marginal cost competitive pricing.

Interviews with hospitals indicate that their pricing practices fit the oligopoly model in another respect: most prices were based on cost-plus calculations. First, the hospitals estimated the cost per unit of output for their numerous services at certain assumed levels of output that were within their capacity to deliver. Then they marked up to these figures to provide for a targeted amount of net income. This practice was rooted in history, since for years Medicare and Medicaid had reimbursed on the basis of costs (Bauerschmidt, 1985). But the practice left hospitals naive about other dimensions of price setting, especially market-oriented factors of price elasticity and measurements of marginal as compared to average costs.

A problem with homogeneous oligopolies that was illustrated in Community A is the effect of heavy promotional activity on raising costs of the entire industry. One hospital's advertising causes others to follow suit, and these several efforts may cancel out any effect on an individual hospital. The total market probably increases little. Yet once every hospital has increased its advertising expenditures no single hospital can reduce this activity without running the risk of losing volume. Thus the cost curves for the industry are pushed beyond the levels that are socially optimal.

IV. SUMMARY

Summing across the three phases, the pattern of evolution was as follows: (1) the emergence of a market orientation by hospitals as the industry moved away from regulation; (2) steady expansion of what the hospitals considered to be their business, to include nonacute and wellness services, with vertical integration and diversification the vehicle for accomplishing this; (3) remarkable change with respect to who was competing with whom, stemming from restructuring of the market toward horizontal concentration and domination by a few rather than continuing open competition among many; (4) a shift in the market from one of competitive consumer choices among physicians and hospitals toward one of competitive choice among health plans; and (5) the beginnings of price dynamics within the context of oligopoly, due primarily to heightened power of corporate and other purchasers.

A striking feature of this evolution was the role of concentration as both a response to increased competition and a vector of change in restructuring the market. Another notable feature was the relationship of vertical and horizontal integrations to each other: Stage I corporate reorganization and limited vertical integration provided the vehicle for horizontal integration in Stage II; then horizontal integration achieved a new critical mass and market dominance, yielding more vertical integration in Stage III.

Finally, we note that of the numerous reasons advanced for mergers in industrial sectors and among hospitals in particular, a singular motivation was pursued in Community A: in an era of increasing competition, the stronger hospitals moved with determination to reduce competition and establish domination. The fundamental motive was market control.

ACKNOWLEDGMENTS

We wish to acknowledge the assistance of the Western Center for Health Planning, San Francisco, and the Bureau of Health Facilities, U.S. Department of Health and Human Services.

REFERENCES

Bauerschmidt, A.D. and P. Jacobs (1985), "Pricing Objectives in Non-Profit Hospitals." *Health Services Research* (June).

Burik, D. (1983), "The Changing Role of Prices: A Framework for Pricing in a Competitive Environment." *Health Care Management Review* 8:2.

Chamberlin, E. (1933), *The Theory of Monopolistic Competition*. Cambridge, MA: Harard University Press.

Starkweather, D. (1981), *Hospital Mergers in the Making*. Ann Arbor, MI: Health Administration Press.

STRATEGIC BEHAVIOR PATTERNS OF SMALL MULTI-INSTITUTIONAL HEALTH ORGANIZATIONS

James W. Begun, Roice D. Luke, T. Alan Jensen, and Lora Hanson Warner

I. INTRODUCTION

The movement toward the restructuring of local hospitals into small multi-institutional health organizations often is overlooked in research on recent health care delivery system developments. About one-third of hospitals in multihospital systems belong to organizations comprised of fewer than eight member hospitals, and small, locally oriented health care systems are the most common type of multihospital system. About 80% of multihospital systems, in both 1982/1983 and 1985, have fewer than eight member hospitals, and about one-half of all systems have either two or three member hospitals. Of the 100 not-for-profit, nonchurch systems, 90 are comprised of two to seven hospitals. Even in the investor-owned segment, 55% of systems are "small" by the same criteria (AHA, 1985). In addition to representing much of multihospital system activity today, small systems serve as a major option for many of the currently freestanding hospitals distributed across the country.

It is likely that patterns of evolution and growth of small systems are distinct from the patterns of development followed by the large investor-owned health and health-related companies. In addition to patterns of strategic

Advances in Health Economics and Health Services Research, Vol. 7, pgs. 195–214.
Copyright © 1987 by JAI Press Inc.
All rights of reproduction in any form reserved.
ISBN: 0-89232-573-9

behavior of the small systems, little is known about their internal structures, cultures, and strategies. Information about the operating characteristics and strategies of small systems should provide clues about the future evolution of the health care industry, as the small systems represent a significant segment of the adaptive activities of hospitals in response to their changing environment.

The purpose of this paper is to delineate the strategic behavior patterns of small multihospital systems. We define small systems as those which range in size from two to seven hospitals. Based upon earlier work (Luke et al., 1985), we first characterize strategic behavior patterns based upon two major dimensions of strategic behavior: a firm's growth orientation and its action orientation. This classification is accomplished with historical and demographic data from a sample of 78 small multihospital systems with 371 member hospitals.

Using questionnaire survey data from 49 of the systems and 169 of the member hospitals, we then characterize the organizational strategies, structure, and culture associated with each strategic behavior pattern. In doing so, we relate a firm's long-term growth orientation and its more recent degree of activity (action orientation) to internal firm characteristics.

Our approach addresses an area neglected in the research literature: the interdependencies among an organization's strategies, structure, and culture. We discuss these interdependencies under the umbrella term *strategic behavior pattern*. We illustrate the interdependencies by locating patterns of strategy, structure, and culture which are associated with specific strategic behavior types.

A second goal of our study is to test the utility of the common differentiation of hospitals (and systems) by ownership. We investigate whether our classification of strategic behavior patterns is more informative than the use of ownership categories, e.g., investor-owned or not-for-profit. The goal is to produce a nomenclature which reflects real differences among organizations. In this case we test the relative ability of ownership categories to differentiate among the strategies, structure, and culture of small multihospital systems.

We expect that a firm's strategic behavior pattern will have significant consequences for its performance. While this relationship is not empirically evaluated in this paper, we hopefully contribute new ways to conceptualize the behavior of organizations so that performance can be better explained, predicted, and controlled.

II. CONCEPTUALIZING STRATEGIC BEHAVIOR PATTERNS: GROWTH AND ACTION ORIENTATIONS

Strategy as a concept is relatively new not only to business management, but to the health care field in particular. Perhaps the most important early work on strategy was produced by Chandler (1962) in his classic study of the evolution and development of American industry. Since that time many have attempted to define and apply the concept of strategy, the result of which has been a rapid expansion in what is called the strategic management literature (see Bracker, 1980; Schendel and Hofer, 1979; and Bourgeois, 1980 for general discussions of the concept of strategy).

A. Growth and Action Orientations

There are not only numerous definitions of strategy, but also many levels at which strategy is applied in organizations. Despite the diversity of typologies available in the literature, most focus either on the key concept underlying a firm's approach to growth or on a firm's pattern of adaptation to changing environments. The first category of typologies is concerned with the primary pathways along which firms grow, which we label a firm's *growth orientation*. While a wide variety of models of growth have been presented in the literature (e.g., Porter, 1980; Ansoff, 1965; Mintzberg and Waters, 1982), there basically are two approaches to achieving growth—by increasing the scale of production of existing activities or by expanding the scope and diversity of activities. Among the most widely recognized typologies of growth are those designed to capture the stages through which firms pass as they grow through time (e.g., Chandler, 1962; Leontiades, 1980). In all of these, major shifts in an organization's pattern of growth are seen to occur when the organization adopts the diversity strategy in preference to the generally less risky pattern of growing through expansion in the scale of dominant business activities.

In characterizing the growth orientations of small multihospital systems, we found that the systems generally were young in their developmental stage, with minimal amounts of non-health-care diversification. Thus the categories of growth orientation presented below for small multihospital systems are defined mainly by the scale of their growth rather than by diversity.

The second major category of typologies of strategic behavior focuses on a firm's pattern of adaptation or reaction to its environment, which we label a firm's *action orientation*. Action orientation is a short-term concept based on Miles and Snow (1978), who argued that organizations possess "theories of action" which are used to select and interpret stimuli from the environment and are reflected in the strategies and ideologies of organizations. Such a firm's reactive pattern could conceivably be altered at any time, as adaptation represents essentially a short-term response to the environment. On the other hand, for such patterns to be strategic rather than tactical, they must be both enduring and significant in terms of their consequences for the long-term development of the firm. These typologies capture a firm's willingness to take risks or its purposefulness in responding to environmental change, regardless of the overall strategies driving its growth.

Below we utilize the best known of these typologies, the Miles et al. (1978) classification of organizations into four strategic types: Defenders, Prospectors, Analyzers, and Reactors. Defender firms concentrate on maintaining stability, control, and efficiency, while Prospector firms seek new product and market opportunities and remain flexible. Analyzers are both stable and dynamic, combining traits of Defenders and Prospectors. Reactor firms adjust to their environment in an inconsistent and unstable pattern, usually performing poorly in the long run as a result.

B.   Empirical Evidence on the Growth and Action Orientations of Small Multihospital Systems

In earlier work (Luke et al., 1985) we analyzed the growth and action orientations of 78 small multihospital systems. Here we review the findings of that study in order to set the stage for identifying the organizational correlates of those strategic behavior patterns.

The sample for the earlier study was selected from the population of 165 nongovernmental multihospital systems of size 2–7 hospitals identified on the American Hospital Association's multihospital system data file for 1982. The sample was selected by nonproportionate random selection within strata based upon four ownership categories (Catholic, investor-owned, church–other, and not-for-profit nonchurch) cross-classified by four size categories (2, 3, 4–5, and 6–7 member hospitals). Investor-owned and church–other systems were proportionately oversampled due to their small numbers in the population, while Catholic systems were undersampled due to their large numbers and the belief that Catholic systems would exhibit more uniformity than other systems. Because investor-owned and church–other systems are larger than average, larger-size systems are overrepresented in the sample.

Based on geographic and telephone survey data collected about the growth and evolution of the 78 systems, we classified the growth and action orientations of the systems. Systems were classified into one of three growth orientations, measured by the size of the parent (originating) hospital in the system, the size of acquired hospitals ("acquired" hospitals included any hospitals joining the system), and the geographic dispersion of the hospitals. Three major models of growth were identified among small multihospital systems: (1) *Investment model*—smaller hospitals (both parent and acquisitions) and wide geographic dispersion; (2) *Local Market model*—large parent, but smaller acquisitions and a low degree of geographic dispersion; (3) *Historical model*—larger hospitals (both parent and acquisitions) and wide geographic dispersion.

Action orientations of the systems were measured by the percentage of hospitals in the system acquired since 1975, the percentage divested since 1981, and the total number of hospitals acquired. Four action orientations were identified in the system sample, as follows: (1) *Prospectors*—large number and percentage of recent acquisitions; (2) *Analyzers*—moderate percentage of recent acquisitions or high percentage if total number was small; (3) *Defenders*—low percentage of recent acquisitions; and (4) *Reactors*—large percentage of recent acquisitions *and* divestitures.

To summarize results of the study, most of the sample (69%) fell into the Local Market growth orientation, with 12% classified as Historical model and 19% as Investment model. Investor-owned and Catholic systems were less likely to be classified as Local Market model systems. Two action orientations were more common in the sample—Analyzers (45%) and Defenders (29%)—with Prospectors comprising 18% of the systems and Reactors 8%. Catholic systems were more likely to be found in the Defender category, while investor-owned systems were more likely to be classified as Prospectors or Reactors. The two dimensions of strategic behavior patterns—growth and action orientations—showed no significant relationship with each other, while each was associated with ownership (as indicated above). We concluded that growth and action orientations were useful ways to classify small-system evolution and growth, and we expect these differences to be reflected in and have implications for the systems' internal processes and structures.

III. ORGANIZATIONAL CORRELATES OF GROWTH AND ACTION ORIENTATIONS: METHODS

In this paper we examine the organizational correlates of strategic behavior patterns by presenting survey data about the structure, strategy, and internal culture of member hospitals within small multihospital systems. The discussion is based upon the position that strategic behavior patterns of firms are determined by firm strategy, structure, and culture. Those organizational dimensions shape the specific response which an organization selects in response to external stimuli (Meyer, 1982; Begun et al., 1985). Responses over time aggregate into what we have described above as growth and action orientations.

A. Questionnaire Survey of Small Multihospital Systems

We contacted the 78 multihospital systems in the sample discussed above by telephone to ask that they participate in a questionnaire survey of system chief executive officers (CEOs) and member hospital CEOs. We received

Table 1.   System Affiliation of Hospital CEO Respondents by System
Ownership and Size in 1982

Ownership of System	System Affiliation of Respondents		Population[a]	
	N	%	N	%
Church-Other	36	22.0	60	9.2
Catholic	41	25.0	282	43.3
Not-for-Profit	76	46.3	249	38.2
Investor-Owned	11	6.7	60	9.2
Total	164	100.0	651	99.9

Size of System	System Affiliation of Respondents		Population[a]	
	N	%	N	%
2 hospitals	15	9.1	180	27.6
3 hospitals	29	17.7	156	24.0
4–5 hospitals	66	40.2	170	26.1
6–7 hospitals	54	32.9	145	22.3
Total	164	99.9	651	100.0

[a]*Source:*   American Hospital Association (1985). Data are for 1982/83.

negative responses or indication that the system was "not really a system"
or was out of business in 16 cases, leaving a sample of 62 systems. Two
different questionnaires were sent to the CEO of each system—a six-page
questionnaire to be completed by the CEO and a two-page background
data questionnaire to be completed by a staff member designated by the
CEO. Six-page questionnaires also were mailed to the 270 member hospitals of the 62 systems, with a cover letter indicating that the corporate
office of the system had agreed to participate in the survey. Data collection
was conducted in June–September 1985.

In this paper we report responses to the hospital CEO survey only. After
one follow-up, responses were received from 169 (63%) of the 270 hospital
CEOs, representing 49 (79%) of the 62 systems in the sample. The distribution of hospital CEO respondents by system size and ownership is
shown in Table 1, along with corresponding population figures. Compared
to the population of hospitals in small systems, the hospital CEOs in our
sample overrepresent not-for-profit systems and underrepresent Catholic
and church–other systems. Smaller systems within the size range also are
underrepresented.

The hospital CEO questionnaire contained questions about the strategies
likely to be pursued by the hospital and its corporate system office, the
degree of centralization of the structure of the system, and the internal

culture of the hospital and the system. As mentioned earlier, these components of the organization should be reflected in and should affect the strategic behavior pattern of the organization. Next, we describe measures for the dimensions of strategy, structure, and culture drawn from the hospital CEO questionnaires.

B. Measurement of Strategy, Structure, and Culture

Because in the design of the questionnaire we sought to obtain multiple indicators of concepts, responses to many of the items on the survey instrument were intercorrelated. Factor analysis was used to simplify the interpretation of these intercorrelations.

Exploratory principal-components factor analysis assumes that variables are linear combinations of underlying factors. The process of factor analysis reveals these basic underlying factors or dimensions for a set of measures and thus reduces observed measures to a minimum number of dimensions which are required to be able to mathematically approximate the correlation matrix of the original variables. A "pure" factor structure is sought where each variable correlates strongly with one underlying dimension and does not correlate with any of the others. This is referred to as orthogonality or independence (Kim and Mueller, 1978). Additionally, the empirical association of a variable with a factor must be corroborated by face validity: all of the variables associated with a factor must logically relate to the same underlying concept (Kaluzny and Veney, 1980).

A separate principal components factor analysis was conducted for each of the three segments of the hospital CEO questionnaire: strategy, structure, and culture. In this way, each of these concepts could be measured in a more parsimonious manner. Also, as an aid to interpretation of the resulting factors, a varimax rotation method was employed in each case. This method clarifies the factor loadings and retains the independence of the factors. The analysis of each section of the questionnaire will be discussed in turn below.

C. Measures of Strategy

Twenty-four items in the questionnaire asked hospital CEOs to rate the importance of specific strategic actions for the future survival of their hospital. Factor analysis reduced the number of items under consideration to 16, and five factors drawn from the 16 items are listed in Table 2. These five dimensions of strategy accounted for 64.0% of the total variance among the 16 items. One factor shown in Table 2, participative control, explained 28% of the variance. The items on this factor relate to increasing physician participation at both the hospital and system level and to allowing more hospital involvement in corporate-level decision making.

Table 2.   Organizational Correlates of Strategic Behavior Patterns:
Measures of Strategy[a]

Demand Expansion

1. Pursue contracts with HMOs or other insurance systems.
2. Pursue contracts with large employers (e.g., wellness programs, industrial medicine, PPOs).

Planning Expansion

1. Increase resources devoted to the marketing function at the individual *hospital* level.
2. Expand clinical services other than traditional inpatient care (e.g., ambulatory, long-term, wellness, substance abuse).
3. Increase resources devoted to the strategic planning function at the individual *hospital* level.

Product/Market Expansion

1. Expand nonclinical areas of hospital service, utilizing existing hospital capabilities (e.g., laundry service, contract management, computer services).
2. Expand nonhealth care businesses (e.g., hotels and restaurants outside of the hospital).
3. Add *nearby* hospitals to the existing system.
4. Add *distant* hosptals to the existing system.

Centralized Control

1. Increase corporate control over individual hospital *operational* decision making.
2. Increase corporate control over individual hospital *strategic* decision making.
3. Increase resources devoted to the marketing function at the *corporate* level.

Participative Control

1. Increase hospital management staff involvement in *corporate* decision making.
2. Implement a more participatory management style.
3. Increase physician involvement in *corporate* decision making.
4. Increase physician involvement in *hospital* decision making.

---

[a]Each concept is measured by the mean of all items, with each item measured on a 1–7 scale rating "the relative importance of the strategy to your *hospital's* long-term survival," with 1 indicating "not important for long-term survival" and 7 indicating "extremely important for long-term survival."

Second, a strategy of centralization at the corporate level was indicated by three items listed in Table 2 under the heading "Centralized Control." These items all reflected a desire by hospital CEOs to increase resources and decision making at the corporate level. This factor explained 12% of the variance.

A strategy of expansion into nontraditional service areas was the third underlying factor, accounting for 10% of the variance. This factor is labeled product/market expansion, as it includes two items reflecting expansion of the multihospital system through the purchase of additional hospitals and two items measuring interest in moving into nonclinical businesses.

A fourth underlying dimension, planning expansion, was indicated by three items relating to greater hospital emphasis on strategic planning, marketing, and new clinical programs. This factor accounted for 8% of the variance.

The final dimension we identified was a strategy of attempting to capture market-based demand through contracting with employers or insurance companies. Two items reflecting the strategy of contracting loaded strongly on this dimension, accounting for 7% of the variance.

The identification of these five factors served to simplify the analysis by reducing the number of items under examination to a set of five dimensions. "Factor-based" scales were then developed using the raw score solution. For each factor, the mean of all items comprising the factor was taken, as the magnitude of the loadings on each variable in the factors was approximately equivalent (Kim and Mueller, 1978; Kaluzny and Veney, 1980).

D. Measures of Strategy

Three underlying dimensions of centralization were revealed by factor analysis of 10 items measuring centralization of decision making in the multihospital system. The resulting scales, constructed from eight different items, are shown in Table 3; the three factors explain 71% of the variance among the eight items.

The first factor identified was composed of three variables which dealt with the appointment of local board members, sale of hospital assets, and change in hospital bylaws. This factor, labeled *centralization of strategic policy*, explained 39% of the variance.

Second, items relating to the centralization of internal hospital operations loaded together on an additional factor, accounting for 19% of the variance. To some extent, these loadings overlapped with a third factor, centralization of CEO control, which was composed of the two items relating to control over the hospital CEOs. The questions concerning appointment and evaluation of the hospital CEOs created a two-item factor which accounted for 13% of the total variance. In the same manner as described in the previous section, factor-based scales were developed for these factors, taking the mean of the raw scores of variables which loaded strongly on each factor. One additional general perceptual measure of centralization, also shown in Table 3, was not included in the factor analysis and was retained as a separate indicator of centralized structure in the multihospital system.

E. Measures of Culture

The survey instrument contained nine beliefs or values for which CEOs rated their predominance in their hospital. The analysis revealed two strong

Table 3.　Organizational Correlates of Strategic Behavior Patterns:
Measures of Structure

Centralization—Strategic[a]

1. Appointment of local board members
2. Sale of hospital assets
3. Change in hospital bylaws

Centralization—CEO[a]

1. Appointment of hospital CEO
2. Performance evaluation of hospital CEO

Centralization—Operating[a]

1. Medical staff privileges
2. Hospital operating budgets
3. Service additions at the hospital level

Centralization—Perceived[b]

To what degree is decision-making power concentrated at the *corporate* organization level?

---

[a]Each concept is measured by the mean of all items, with each item measured on a 1–7 scale in response to the following question: "For each type of decision, how much influence does the *corporate office* of this multihospital system have?" Here 1 indicates "no influence" and 7 indicates "a great deal of influence."
[b]Measured on a 1–7 scale, with 1 indicating "low degree" and 7 indicating "high degree."

factors using five of the items: the belief in a business/profit orientation and the belief in a community service orientation. Table 4 gives items comprising the two factors. Factor 1, profit value, accounted for 33% of the variance, while Factor 2, service value, explained 22% of the variance among the five items.

Again, factor-based scales were developed measuring the predominance of profit and service values in the hospitals. Finally, three single-item measures of conflict between member hospitals and the corporate office of the multihospital system were used as indicators of the internal culture of the system. They also are shown in Table 4.

IV.　ORGANIZATIONAL CORRELATES OF GROWTH AND ACTION ORIENTATIONS: FINDINGS

Mean values for the five measures of strategy, four measures of structure, and five measures of culture used in this study are reported in Table 5.

First, we will describe the strategies which the system members would like to pursue. Hospital CEOs in this sample of systems exhibit greatest interest (a mean rating of 5.8 on a 7-point scale) in the strategy of "planning

Table 4. Organizational Correlates of Strategic Behavior Patterns:
Measures of Culture

Profit Value[a]

1. The belief that health care is primarily a business
2. The belief that a profit motivation leads to increased organizational effectiveness
3. The belief that competition in health care delivery is superior to regulation

Service Value[a]

1. The belief that health care is a right for all
2. The belief that hospitals are primarily community service organizations

Mission Conflict[b]

To what degree is there conflict between the *missions* of member hospitals and the corporate organization?

Strategy Conflict[b]

To what degree is there conflict between the *strategies* of member hospitals and the corporate organization?

Loyalty Conflict[b]

To what degree do member hospital CEOs have conflicting *loyalties* between their hospitals and the corporate organization?

---

[a]Each concept is measured by the mean of all items, with each item measured on a 1–7 scale rating "the extent to which the following beliefs are *predominant* in your hospital," with 1 indicating "not at all predominant" and 7 indicating "extremely predominant."
[b]Measured on a 1–7 scale, with 1 indicating "low degree" and 7 indicating "high degree."

expansion," which is reflective of mainstream hospital adaptive behavior today—improving planning and marketing capabilities and expanding clinically related specialty services other than inpatient care. Also rated as very important (5.5) is the strategy of "demand expansion" through the pursuit of large-scale contracts. "Participative control" is rated third highest (5.0) among the types of strategies to pursue in the future, and it is the last strategy rated above the midpoint of the scale from "not important" to "extremely important." Rated lowest were the strategy of centralizing decision making (4.0) and the strategy of product/market expansion (3.5). Hospital CEOs perceived that it was of little importance to their long-term survival, then, to centralize decision making more at the corporate offices of their systems or to expand system size through the acquisition of new hospitals or development of nonclinical products and services.

On the dimension of internal culture, hospital CEOs ascribe about equal weight to the predominance of profit (4.9) and service (5.1) values in their hospitals. Levels of conflict between member hospitals and corporate offices in small multihospital systems are perceived to be low to moderate, with mean values on questions measuring the degree of conflict over strat-

Table 5.   Descriptive Statistics for Strategy, Structure, and Culture
Measures, Based on Member Hospital CEO Responses[a]

	Mean	*Standard Deviation*
Strategy (Hospital)		
Demand Expansion	5.49	1.35
Planning Expansion	5.82	.93
Product/Market Expansion	3.53	1.23
Centralized Control	4.04	1.34
Participative Control	5.01	1.05
Structure		
Centralization—Strategic	5.45	1.51
Centralization—CEO	6.31	1.10
Centralization—Operating	4.90	1.37
Centralization—Perceived	4.40	1.58
Culture (Hospital)		
Profit Value	4.94	1.02
Service Value	5.07	1.21
Mission Conflict	2.59	1.58
Strategy Conflict	3.25	1.58
Loyalty Conflict	3.43	1.80

[a]N ranges from 166 to 168.

egy (3.3), mission (2.6) and CEO loyalty (3.4) all falling below the midpoint of a 1–7 scale from low to high.

Corporate office influence on the appointment and evaluation of hospital CEOs is reported to be very high (6.3), as is corporate influence over hospital strategic policies (5.5). Corporate control of operating policies is rated as moderately high (4.9). Despite this evidence that decision making is fairly centralized, hospital CEOs perceive only a moderate (4.4) degree of concentration of power at the corporate level, perhaps because the questionnaire items reflected less common, higher-level policy decisions.

Based on member hospital CEO responses, then, we would characterize small multihospital systems as follows: profit and service values coexist; there is strong agreement among members about the system's mission and strategy; there is moderately to highly centralized control over decision making; and hospitals perceive the need to continue to capture demand through the pursuit of clinical services other than inpatient care, within their service areas. Some hint of dissension with centralized corporate control may be reflected in the member hospital CEOs' preference for more participative management in the system (relative to greater central-

Table 6. Mean Values of Strategy, Structure, and Culture Measures by
Action Orientation of System[a]

	Action Orientation of System		
	Defender	*Analyzer*	*Prospector*
Strategy (Hospital)			
Demand Expansion	5.6	5.5	5.4
Planning Expansion	6.1	5.8	5.7
Product/Market Expansion	3.9	3.5	3.4
Centralized Control	4.2	4.1	3.8
Participative Control	5.1	4.9	5.2
Structure			
Centralization—Strategic**	6.1	5.6	4.7
Centralization—CEO	6.1	6.3	6.5
Centralization—Operating	5.0	4.9	4.9
Centralization—Perceived	4.3	4.3	4.7
Culture			
Profit Value	4.8	5.0	4.9
Service Value**	5.4	5.0	4.8
Mission Conflict**	2.3	2.4	3.1
Strategy Conflict**	3.2	3.0	3.8
Loyalty Conflict**	3.4	3.2	4.0

[a]Total N ranges from 166 to 168, with 34–36 Defenders, 84–85 Analyzers, and 46–48 Prospectors.
**Significant differences between two or more categories exist, based upon Duncan's multiple range test,
alpha = .05.

ization of decision making at the corporate level) and the low rating as-
signed to product/market expansion strategies.

A. The Organizational Correlates of Action Orientations

Next we assess the usefulness of the concept of action orientation in
depicting internal strategy, structure, and culture differences among small
multihospital systems. Table 6 gives means values of the measures of strategy, structure, and culture for hospitals belonging to Defender, Analyzer,
and Prospector multihospital systems. No hospitals belonging to the fourth
category of action orientation, Reactor systems, appear in the table, as
most hospitals belonging to those systems in 1982 had been divested by
1985 and thus were not in our survey sample. Means are compared across
categories for significant differences using Duncan's multiple-range test.

From Table 6 we conclude that systems' action orientations are strongly
associated with the internal culture of the system. Prospector firms, in
particular, have distinguishing cultural traits. On all three measures of

conflict, Prospector systems rate significantly higher than Defender and Analyzer systems. Recalling that Prospector systems are defined by a high degree of recent acquisition activity, these findings of lower internal cohesion are reasonable. Prospector systems also exhibit a significantly lower community service orientation than Defender systems. Defender systems are defined by less recent acquisition activity, and this inactivity may to some degree reflect a reluctance to sacrifice a traditional community service orientation.

Measures of internal culture in Analyzer systems fall between the Defender and Prospector categories on the service value dimension, while closely resembling Defender systems on the three measures of conflict— strategy, mission, and loyalty. Thus Analyzer systems seem to preserve high levels of internal cohesion while operating actively in the acquisition arena.

System action orientations fail to aid in identifying differences in the types of strategy sought by member hospital CEOs, as no significant differences appear across action orientations for the strategies listed in Table 6. One pattern which seems apparent, however, is that Defender systems rate all of the strategies except one (participative control) as more important to their future survival than do Analyzer and Prospector systems. It may be that Defender systems perceive a more precarious position for themselves, and thus a greater need to be active in the strategic arena. Consistent with this argument, Prospector system hospitals rate all of the strategies except participative control lower in importance than do Defender and Analyzer system hospitals.

Turning to measures of centralization, system action orientations are predictive only of centralization of strategic policy, as Defenders and Analyzers report significantly greater corporate control of strategic policy than do Prospectors. Prospector systems apparently are satisfied with this lower degree of corporate control of strategic policy, given their low rating of centralized control as a future strategy.

To summarize, a system's action orientation is particularly useful in distinguishing among elements of the internal cultures of small multihospital systems. Prospector systems, in particular, are differentiated from Defender systems. Defender systems are more centralized and exhibit more internal cohesion, apparently avoiding the internal turmoil associated with recent changes in composition which Prospector systems have experienced.

B.   The Organizational Correlates of Growth Orientations

Growth orientation, the long-term pattern of evolution of the system, is of some value in distinguishing the strategies for the future envisioned by member hospital CEOs, as portrayed in Table 7. Historical model firms,

Table 7. Mean Values of Strategy, Structure, and Culture Measures by Growth Orientation of System[a]

	Growth Orientation of System		
	Local Market	Historical	Investment
Strategy (Hospital)			
Demand Expansion**	5.5	5.9	5.2
Planning Expansion**	5.8	6.3	5.7
Product/Market Expansion	3.5	3.9	3.4
Centralized Control	4.0	4.2	4.0
Participative Control	5.1	5.0	4.8
Structure			
Centralization—Strategic	5.3	6.0	5.5
Centralization—CEO	6.4	6.1	6.2
Centralization—Operating**	5.0	4.2	4.9
Centralization—Perceived	4.5	4.3	3.9
Culture			
Profit Value	5.0	5.0	4.8
Service Value	5.1	5.0	5.2
Mission Conflict	2.6	2.5	2.5
Strategy Conflict	3.3	3.0	3.2
Loyalty Conflict	3.6	3.2	3.0

[a]Total N ranges from 166 to 168, with 113–155 Local Market, 22 Historical, and 30–31 Investment.
**Significant differences between two or more categories exist, based upon Duncan's multiple range test, alpha = .05.

those characterized by widely dispersed large hospitals, are significantly more interested in strategies of demand and planning expansion than are Investment model firms, those composed of widely dispersed small hospitals. Historical model firms also exhibit greater interest in product/market expansion, although the difference is not statistically signficant. CEOs in each of the three types of systems assign approximately the same rating to the importance of centralization and participation strategies. Historical model firms, then, express the desire to be most active in the strategic arena. One might argue that hospitals in these firms have the potential to be very active in local markets, due to their size, and that they perhaps have been handicapped because they have no system "partners" at the local market level. Thus, autonomous strategic action is more critical to their future survival than is the case for Local Market systems and is more feasible than is the case for the smaller Investment model system hospitals.

Growth orientations are associated with the measure of centralization dealing with hospital operating decisions, as Historical system hospitals report significantly less corporate control of hospital operating decisions than do Local Market and Investment model hospitals. This is consistent with the image of Historical model firms being driven less by local market or financial conditions than the other two types of firms. While not significantly different, Historical model firms do report a *higher* degree of strategic policy centralization, perhaps reflecting control by mission or service orientation at the top level.

Long-term patterns of evolution fail to associate with internal cultural measures, as portrayed in the lower part of Table 7. No significant differences among the Local Market, Historical, and Investment models emerge on the measures of system and hospital culture.

We conclude that past growth orientations are moderately associated with a firm's strategies. The failure of the growth orientation to distinguish among current cultural and structural characteristcs of systems may reflect the fact that growth orientations measure past actions, over a long period of time, while our measures of strategy, structure, and culture reflect recent and future activities.

V. THE ORGANIZATIONAL CORRELATES OF OWNERSHIP

What does ownership tell us about firm structure, strategy, and culture? In this section we examine more closely exactly what ownership tells us about hospitals in small multihospital systems.

From Table 8 it is evident that ownership is highly correlated with facets of both system structure and culture. Regarding structure, Catholic systems are significantly less centralized than other systems on three of the four centralization measures. On the fourth measure, centralization of strategic policy, Catholic systems rank *highest* (although they are not significantly different). These findings are consistent with corporate guidance of Catholic systems at the mission/policy level, reflected in the sponsorship relationship between many Catholic orders and their affiliated hospitals, but little interference in more operational activities of the hospitals. The reverse is true for the investor-owned systems, which rank lowest on corporate control of strategic policy but highest on the operational and general perception measures of centralization. Not-for-profit and church–other systems fall between the Catholic vs. investor-owned extremes.

Ownership distinguishes among four of the five measures of system culture. Hospitals in investor-owned systems claim a significantly higher presence of a belief in profit making, while hospitals in Catholic systems display a stronger belief in community service values and a less pervasive belief in profit making. Conflict between member hospitals and corporate offices

Table 8. Mean Values of Strategy, Structure, and Culture Measures by Ownership of System[a]

| | Ownership of System | | | |
	Church–Other	Catholic	Not-for-Profit	Investor-Owned
Strategy (Hospital)				
Demand Expansion	5.2	5.8	5.4	5.6
Planning Expansion	5.9	6.0	5.7	5.7
Product/Market Expansion	3.8	3.8	3.2	3.2
Centralized Control	4.1	4.0	4.0	4.0
Participative Control	5.1	5.0	4.9	5.1
Structure				
Centralization–Strategic	5.5	5.8	5.3	5.1
Centralization—CEO**	6.4	5.8	6.5	6.7
Centralization—Operating**	5.2	4.4	4.9	5.5
Centralization–Perceived**	4.4	3.8	4.6	5.0
Culture				
Profit Value**	4.9	4.7	5.0	5.4
Service Value**	4.6	5.7	5.0	4.9
Mission Conflict**	2.6	2.3	2.6	3.5
Strategy Conflict**	3.1	3.1	3.3	4.1
Loyalty Conflict	3.4	3.4	3.4	3.5

[a]Total N ranges from 161 to 164, with 35–36 Church–Other, 42–43 Catholic, 72–74 Not-for-Profit, and 11 Investor-Owned.
**Significant differences between two or more categories exist, based upon Duncan's multiple range test, alpha = .05.

over hospital mission and strategy is significantly higher in investor-owned systems. Catholic systems exhibit low degrees of internal conflict.

No significant differences among system ownership categories are evident in hospital CEOs' opinions about future survival strategies.

In summary, ownership categories seem to have strong implications for firm structure and culture. Roughly, Catholic-owned systems exhibit decentralized control at the operating level and a high degree of adherence to a service value and congruence about strategy and mission among members. Investor-owned systems control hospital operations to a greater degree and have relatively higher degrees of internal conflict and adherence to profit-making values. We speculate that the presence of conflict and predominance of the profit value in investor-owned systems may be related due to the historical antipathy for profit-making values in hospitals.

VI. CONCLUSIONS

We have described the strategy, structure, and internal culture of small multihospital systems. The picture which emerges is one of relative uniformity of strategic outlook: small-system hospitals plan to pursue strategies of market control through development and marketing of clinically related services and contracts for clinical services. Member hospitals are interested in greater rather than lesser participation in system decision making and are least interested in system growth or expansion into non-health-care businesses. Corporate control of the hospitals is viewed to be moderate to high, but this does not result in high levels of conflict between member hospitals and their corporate offices. Both profit-making and community service values are perceived to be pervasive in small-system hospitals.

We have tested the linkage between action orientation, growth orientation, ownership and measures of strategy, structure, and culture in the systems. Generally, action orientations are predictive of internal culture, with hospitals in Defender systems showing low degrees of conflict and an emphasis on service values. Greater involvement in the strategic arena, then, may sacrifice internal cohesion and traditionally shared values, as reflected in the higher levels of conflict reported by Prospector system hospitals. Growth orientations are somewhat useful in predicting hospital strategy, with Historical system hospitals exhibiting the greatest interest in the "mainstream" strategies of competing through the provision of clinical services. Ownership, finally, is associated with structural and cultural variables, with Catholic system hospitals and investor-owned system hospitals standing generally at ends of a continuum on centralization, service and profit values, and intrasystem conflict. Ownership proves to be a relatively strong predictive concept based on the findings here. This is consistent with an argument that firms are "imprinted" by their initial founding, particularly in their internal structure and culture, and that these original structures and values have enduring effects.

Surprisingly, none of the classification schemes was particularly useful in explaining future strategies of small-system hospitals. This may be due to relative homogeneity across the industry regarding perceived strategic options as measured in this study.

Regarding linkages among strategy, structure, and culture, there is some suggestion in the findings that small multihospital system structure and culture are related, as highly centralized systems seem to be characterized by greater internal conflict. Potential linkages between strategy and firm structure and culture probably are attenuated by the fact that the strategy measures used here are prospective, while the culture and structure measures are current or retrospective.

These findings are constrained by the nature of the data, which are collected from a sample in which not-for-profit and church–other system hospitals are overrepresented (see Table 1). Because the data are cross-sectional, it is difficult to speculate on the direction of causality in some relationships, e.g., whether centralization causes more conflict or more conflict causes more centralization. Additionally, the hospital characteristics are based on the responses of a single respondent per organization, and different numbers/proportions of member hospitals are represented in different systems. Finally, several variables which might affect hospital strategy, structure, and culture, most notably market characteristics and system size, were not included in the analyses described above.

Future research activity with these data will compare hospital CEO perceptions with *corporate* CEO perceptions of system strategy, structure, and culture and thus will provide additional evidence about the nature of the relationship between member hospitals and corporate offices in small multihospital systems. In addition, financial performance data are being collected in order to test the performance implications of the different strategic behavior patterns exhibited by these small systems.

ACKNOWLEDGMENT

Partial support for this project was provided by a grant from the W.K. Kellogg Foundation.

REFERENCES

American Hospital Association (1985), *Data Book on Multihospital Systems, 1980–1985*. Chicago: American Hospital Association.

Ansoff, H. Igor (1965), *Corporate Strategy: An Analytic Approach to Growth and Expansion*. New York: McGraw-Hill.

Begun, James W., T. Alan Jensen, and Roice D. Luke (1985), "Action Orientations of Health Care Organizations: Patterns of Structure, Strategy and Culture." Paper presented at the Annual Meeting of the Academy of Management, San Diego, August 11–14.

Bourgeois, L.J. (1980), "Strategy and Environment: A Conceptual Integration." *Academy of Management Review* 5:25–29.

Bracker, J. (1980), "The Historical Development of the Strategic Management Concept." *Academy of Management Review* 5:219–224.

Chandler, Alfred D. (1962), *Strategy and Structure*. Cambridge, MA: MIT Press.

Kaluzny, Arnold and James E. Veney (1980), *Health Service Organizations: A Guide to Research and Assessment*. Berkeley, CA: McCutchan.

Kim, Jae-On and Charles W. Mueller (1978), *Factor Analysis: Statistical Methods and Practical Issues*. Beverly Hills, CA: Sage.

Leontiades, Milton (1980), *Strategies for Diversification and Change*. Boston: Little, Brown.

Luke, Roice D., James W. Begun, and T. Alan Jensen (1985), "Determinants of Evolution and Growth in Complex Hospital Systems." Paper presented at the Annual Meeting of the American Public Health Association, Washington, DC, November 20.

Meyer, Alan D. (1982), "Adapting to Environmental Jolts." *Administrative Science Quarterly* 27(4):515–537.

Miles, Raymond E. and Charles C. Snow (1978), *Organizational Strategy, Structure, and Process*. New York: McGraw-Hill.

Miles, Raymond E., Charles C. Snow, Alan D. Meyer, and Henry J. Coleman, Jr. (1978), "Organizational Strategy, Structure, and Process." *Academy of Management Review* 3(July):546–562.

Mintzberg, Henry and J.A. Waters (1982), "Tracking Strategy in an Entrepreneurial Firm." *Academy of Management Journal* 25:465–499.

Porter, Michael E. (1980), *Competitive Strategy*. New York: Free Press.

Schendel, D.E. and C.W. Hofer (1979), *Strategic Management: A New View of Business Policy and Planning*. New York: McGraw-Hill.

COMMENTS ON BEHAVIOR AND PERFORMANCE

Dan Ermann

All the papers in Part II of this volume examine multihospital systems and their interaction with the rest of the delivery system. They are interesting and important because they provide insights on issues that are largely unexplored. While I will concentrate my comments on the paper by Begun and his colleagues, I have a few introductory notes about two other papers and their contributions to our understanding of the changing health care delivery system.

In recent years, much has been written regarding the ongoing revolution in the health care market. However, there are some issues which have been largely ignored by the research community. For example, we have only recently begun to understand how multihospital systems perform and the importance of differentiating between systems with different characteristics, e.g., differing strategies and organizational structure. Begun et al. examine small systems (with between two and seven hospitals) in an initial attempt at understanding this segment of the industry. Barrett and Campbell, on the other hand, present preliminary case study findings concerning the interaction between physician behavior and the goals and ac-

Advances in Health Economics and Health Services Research, Vol. 7, pgs. 215–217.
Copyright © 1987 by JAI Press Inc.
All rights of reproduction in any form reserved.
ISBN: 0-89232-573-9

tions of a large multihospital system. The paper by Starkweather and Carman examines hospital competitive behavior in three different California communities.

The paper by Starkweather and Carman attempts to explain hospital behavior and strategies by comparing the hospital markets in the three California communities and relating this to the "efficiency and effectiveness of the hospital industry." A case study approach may currently be the best way to examine hospital behavior. This area is still exploratory in nature, and until we have refined our analytical tools and developed necessary data sets, we should rely on case study information to guide our thinking. The authors, however, should be careful in inferring any causal relationships. They must remember that system changes (such as the MediCal contracting program) do not have an immediate impact on hospital operations. The authors are sensitive to the strengths and weaknesses of the case approach, and it would be helpful to provide the reader with details on such issues as the sampling criteria for the choice of hospitals to study. While it is possible to develop hypotheses and even present preliminary findings, we must be very careful in generalizing to other settings.

Barrett and Campbell study the relationship between hospitals and physicians in their paper. Again, this is an area of much interest and conjecture, but little empirical information. The case study approach used seems appropriate, and we can learn from a study of two hospitals. The findings suggest that hospitals interact with their attending physicians differently depending on a myriad of factors, such as the hospital corporate structure and physician characteristics, e.g., age, sex, and specialty. The authors point out that physicians are not a homogeneous group and that hospital strategies must be tailored to the individual physicians practicing at a hospital. With this important finding in mind, Barrett and Campbell remind us that it is difficult to generalize to other Hospital Corporation of America hospitals or to other for-profit system institutions.

The paper by Begun and his colleagues examines the growth strategies of small multi-institutional health organizations (MHOs)—those with less than eight member hospitals. This is an area which has been largely ignored by researchers. Most of the attention is the literature has focused on large systems. Begun et al. point out that of all multihospital systems in 1985, about 80% were small.

This paper presents survey findings based on responses from 169 hospital chief executive officers (CEOs) representing 49 systems. The questions dealt with the CEOs' perceptions of the MHOs strategies (e.g., market expansion), structure (e.g., centralized vs. decentralized decision making), and culture (e.g., importance of profit vs. community service). Again there are problems in generalizing from the results. In this study the relatively low response rate, which overrepresents some forms of hospitals and underrepresents others, may introduce response bias. Also, because of the nature of the multihospital industry, many (if not most) hospital administrators are more concerned with their individual facility than with the whole system. Thus we cannot assume that hospital administrators' perceptions or beliefs, as captured by the survey, are representative of their systems actual operation.

I was unsure of the theoretical basis for some of the models presented, e.g., the three models of growth (Investment model, Local Market model, and Historical model) and the four action models (Prospectors, Analyzers, Defenders, and Reactors). The last four models are determined by time and may only signify the stage of a system at any point in time. More information on the rationale for the models would assist the reader in interpreting the results.

The findings concerning which strategies system members would like to pursue is interesting. It is difficult, however, to weigh the relative importance of CEO answers; i.e., how much more important is a score of 5.0 than one of 4.0? Although some of the differences were statistically significant, the findings should be interpreted according to their policy significance; i.e., are observed differences meaningful in a practical sense? I found this paper worthwhile in exploring new areas, but requiring additional information which would help in interpreting the results.

PART III:

ANTITRUST ISSUES

ANTITRUST TREATMENT OF NONPROFIT AND FOR-PROFIT HOSPITAL MERGERS

Roger D. Blair and James M. Fesmire

I. INTRODUCTION

Containing increases in health care expenditures has been a matter of growing concern in the United States. The percentage of gross national product devoted to national health expenditures rose to 10.5% in 1982 from 7.9% a decade earlier. The portion of health care expenditures devoted to hospital care in 1982 was 42% according to John Miles (1984; 255). The National Health Planning and Resources Development Act of 1974 was an attempt to deal with these cost increases through regulation and control. More recently, there has been a growing feeling that perhaps competitive forces should play a larger role in bringing about efficiency and cost containment. Recent years have seen a rapid growth in the for-profit hospital sector and, along with it, an increase in merger activity.

Nonprofit hospitals presently dominate the industry and it seems they may enjoy exemption from the merger provisions of Clayton 7. This paper will argue that if economic efficiency and consumer welfare are the primary goals of the antitrust laws,[1] then this extension of preferential treatment makes little sense. It will not address the broader question of what overall

Advances in Health Economics and Health Services Research, Vol. 7, pgs. 219–244.
Copyright © 1987 by JAI Press Inc.
All rights of reproduction in any form reserved.
ISBN: 0-89232-573-9

policy should be toward mergers in the hospital industry. The more limited purpose is instead to show that whatever policy posture is adopted toward hospital mergers, whether it be hostile or permissive, preferential treatment toward nonprofit hospitals can only result in a reduction in efficiency and consumer welfare.

We first look at the antitrust framework of merger policy, finishing with a discussion of the possible loophole for nonprofit mergers. Next, we look at the possible motives for mergers and analyze their efficiency effects. Then, judicial and U.S. Department of Justice attitudes toward horizontal mergers are explored with emphasis on attitudes toward efficiency considerations. Next, the peculiarities of the health care market are examined briefly and the performance of nonprofit hospitals is examined. Finally, the effect of disparate treatment of nonprofit and for-profit hospitals under Clayton 7 is analyzed, and it is concluded that preferential treatment of nonprofit hospitals would have negative effects for efficiency and consumer welfare.

II. ANTITRUST FRAMEWORK

Our antitrust arsenal is comprised of the Sherman Act of 1890, the Clayton Act of 1914, and the Federal Trade Commission Act of 1914. Each statute can be used to challenge mergers.

A. Historical Background[2]

Following the Civil War, there was an extended period of agrarian discontent due to the general unprofitability of farming. At the same time that agricultural prices were low, the railroads seemed to be charging "all that the traffic would bear," as were the grain elevator operators. In addition, tariffs, patents, and local monopoly power combined to raise the prices of farm equipment. In response, the farm community formed political pressure groups to do something about monopoly

At about the same time, public sentiment generally became hostile toward the business community due to a steady revelation of (1) questionable business practices involving predation and political corruption, and (2) the formation of price fixing rings, pools, and trusts which raised prices to consumers generally. Ultimately, this culminated in the passage of the Sherman Act in 1890.

The Sherman Act provided vague and general prohibitions of trade restraints and monopolization. The statute's lack of specificity implicitly left it to the judiciary to develop the law of antitrust. As the courts set about their business of interpreting the Sherman Act, a certain uneasiness developed. Many people feared judicial discretion. Some felt that the judiciary would be too severe, while others worried that it would be too lax. In response to a demand for greater specificity and less judicial discretion, Congress enacted the Clayton Act of 1914. In the same year, Congress also passed the Federal Trade Commission Act, which established an agency specifically designed to implement and enforce the antitrust laws.

B. Merger Provisions

Section 2 of the Sherman Act [15 U.S.C. §2(1982)] deals with market structure in a remedial fashion:

> Every person who shall monopolize, or attempt to monopolize, or combine or conspire with any other person or persons, to monopolize any part of the trade or commerce among the several States, or with foreign nations, shall be deemed guilty of a felony . . .

Although this provision of the antitrust laws has been used in merger cases, the standards for proving antitrust liability under Section 2 are fairly severe (Blair and Kaserman, 1985). As a result, most challenges to mergers are filed under Section 7 of the Clayton Act [15 U.S.C. §18(1982)]. In contrast to the remedial nature of the Sherman Act, Section 7 of the Clayton Act, which was amended by the Celler–Kefauver Act of 1950, provides a preventive measure.

When Congress passed the Clayton Act, it did so in order "to arrest the creation of trusts, conspiracies and monopolies in their incipiency and before consummation" (Senate Report, 1914, p. 1). It is clear that the Clayton Act's prohibition of certain mergers was intended to be preventive. Unfortunately, the original language of Section 7 specifically prohibited the acquisition of a rival firm's stock, but was silent on asset acquisitions. This, of course, provided a giant loophole since there is no economic difference in these alternative avenues to consolidation. Following decades of singular ineffectiveness in coping with anticompetitive mergers, the Celler–Kefauver Act closed the asset loophole. Now, Section 7 provides

> [t]hat no person engaged in commerce or in any activity affecting commerce shall acquire, directly or indirectly, the whole or any part of the stock or other share capital and no person subject to the jurisdiction of the Federal Trade Commission shall acquire the whole or any part of the assets of another person engaged also in commerce or in any activity affecting commerce, where in any line of commerce or in any activity affecting commerce in any section of the country, the effect of such acquisition may be substantially to lessen competition, or to tend to create a monopoly.

There are several things that we should note about this language. First, a plaintiff need only show that a merger *may* have the proscribed effect. Thus, the language of Section 7 facilitates challenging a merger where a substantial lessening of competition or tendency toward monopoly is only a *possibility*.[3] In other words, no actual adverse competitive impact need be shown. As a result, Section 7 can be useful in preventing the sort of market structure that is most conducive to collusive behavior or single-firm dominance. Second, as the statute now reads, Section 7 applies to all types of mergers: horizontal, vertical, and conglomerate, Finally, we should note that the proscribed effect on competition must be related to a "line of commerce" in a "section of the country"; i.e., a product market and a geographic market must be defined in order to evaluate the competitive impact.

C. Loophole for Nonprofit Hospitals

There is an apparent loophole in the Clayton Act for mergers of nonprofit hospitals.[4] Section 7 of the Clayton Act applies to nonprofit as well as for-profit hospitals when *stock* acquisitions are involved. When *asset* acquisitions are involved, however, the acquiring party must be "subject to the jurisdiction of the Federal Trade Commission." Now, the FTC Act applies to persons, partnerships, and corporations [15 U.S.C. §45(a)(2)]. In Section 4 of the FTC Act, *corporation* is defined to include any business entity that is "organized to carry on business for its own profit or that of its members" (15 U.S.C. §44). Due to this limited definition of *corporation* in the FTC Act, asset acquisitions involving nonprofit hospitals *may* be exempt from Clayton Act coverage.

We cannot be certain that nonprofit hospitals are exempt from Section 7 coverage because there has not been a case brought to settle the issue. If nonprofit hospitals escape antitrust scrutiny due to the limited definition of *corporation* in the FTC Act, this is an important loophole because the nonprofit hospital is the modal organizational form in the industry. Consequently, this exemption could apply to a large number of hospital mergers.

III. MOTIVES FOR MERGERS

There are many specific incentives for mergers. Based upon the standard theory of the firm, however, the main motivation for a merger is to enhance profits. Since profit is the difference between total revenue and total cost, profits will rise whenever revenues increase, costs decrease, or both. A merger can yield greater revenues when market power is enhanced and noncompetitive pricing results. On the other hand, costs may decrease when operating efficiency is improved due to the exploitation of scale economies. We shall examine each of these in turn.

A. Merging for Market Power[5]

The major antitrust concern with horizontal mergers centers on those mergers that enhance market power. These mergers increase profits by enabling the industry to price at noncompetitive levels.

Merging to Monopoly. In the limit, a merger among all the firms in an industry can be seen as a perfect form of collusion. There can be no cheating and no disputes over territories, customers, or market shares because a single-firm monopoly will have resulted. The only remaining difficulty is controlling entry, which will prove to be quite difficult due to the presence of excess profits. More importantly, however, merging to monopoly will seldom succeed due to the profit incentives for firms to remain outside the consolidation.

In merging to monopoly, it will become increasingly more expensive to acquire independent firms. This can be seen in Figure 1, where the average and marginal cost curves are labeled AC and MC, respectively, and the *proportional* demand function and the associated marginal revenue are d and mr. Prior to the merger activity, each firm would have produced the competitive output of q_1 and sold it at the competitive price of P_1. In the short run, the ultimate goal of a merger to monopoly in this industry is to have each plant producing q_2. As a result of the reduced production, price would rise to P_2 and excess profits per plant would be $(P_2 - C_2)q_2$. But the value to the independent firm if it refuses to merge will be much larger than that. If the firm depicted in Figure 1 were to remain independent, then it could act as a price taker and view P_2 as its marginal revenue function. As a price taker, the optimal output for this firm would be q_3 where its marginal cost equals P_2. Its profit in this case is much larger than $(P_2 - C_2)q_2$. Thus, it is more profitable to remain outside the consolidation. In order to convince the recalcitrant firm that merger is in its best interest, the merged firm may have to resort to some predatory behavior. An alternative would be to simply ignore those firms that refuse to sell out. The optimal price and output would then follow the familiar dominant-firm model. If there are not too many firms outside the consolidation, the results will still be noncompetitive.

Merging to Oligopoly. Due to the problem just mentioned and a host of other things, mergers may stop short of monopoly. In other words, we may witness merging to oligopoly. The concern with oligopoly is confused by the fact that we have a somewhat shaky understanding of what happens in oligopolistic industries. Nonetheless, most of the concern centers on noncompetitive pricing. We know that price fixing leads to higher profits for the colluders. We also know that collusion is much more likely to be

Figure 1

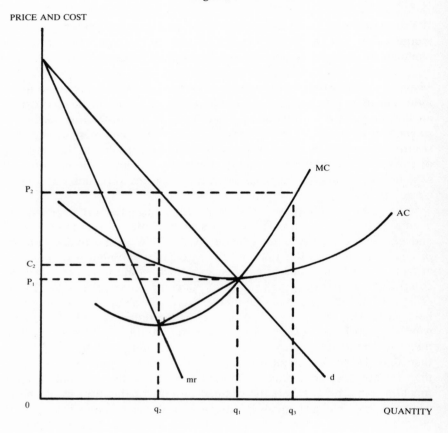

successful with a small number of firms.[6] This results from the fact that the costs of reaching an agreement, implementing that agreement, and policing and enforcing the agreement are lower the smaller the number of firms.

When mergers in an industry result in oligopoly, the firms recognize their mutual interdependence. Some people feel that overt collusion is not even necessary under these circumstances. Instead, the firms may achieve the results of overt collusion through tacit understandings. In the most extreme case, we could have monopoly pricing without any overt collusion.[7]

B. Merging for Improved Efficiency

For mergers that result in market power without any increase in efficiency, the welfare effects are easy to assess—at least on a conceptual level. Since prices rise and output falls, these mergers should not be permitted because consumer welfare is impaired. But some mergers are induced by a quest for greater profits through reduced costs. If such mergers occur, there will be excess profits at least in the short run. In this instance, however, the excess profits are desirable because greater efficiency is properly rewarded. Moreover, these excess profits will provide the correct signals to other firms. Unless some entry barrier is erected, entry of new firms or further mergers within the industry will restore competition in the industry. The welfare results of such a merger are unambiguously positive. These cost reductions reflect real cost savings for society. This effect may be so strong that welfare can be improved as the result of efficiencies, even when prices are increased as a result of an increase in concentration.[8] We shall consider such a case in Figure 2.

Industry demand is shown as D and average costs prior to the merger are AC_1.[9] Assuming that competition prevails initially, price would reflect the costs of production and would be equal to P_1 (and AC_1).[10] Suppose that a merger yields a reduction in costs due to production or promotional efficiencies that save resources. As a result, the average cost of production falls from AC_1 to AC_2. At the same time, market power increases and price rises from P_1 to P_2.[11] Due to the price rise, there is clearly a net welfare loss, which is equal to $\frac{1}{2}(P_2 - P_1)(Q_1 - Q_2)$, or area A_1[12] which must be compared to rectangle A_2, which represents the reduced costs of producing the output Q_2. This cost saving is equal to the area $(AC_1 - AC_2)Q_2$.[13] If the goal of antitrust policy is the maximization of consumer welfare, then the issue is clear. If the cost savings represented by A_2 outweigh the deadweight loss represented by A_1, then consumer welfare is enhanced and the merger should be permitted. If A_1 is larger than A_2, then consumer welfare is reduced and the merger should be proscribed.[14]

Figure 2

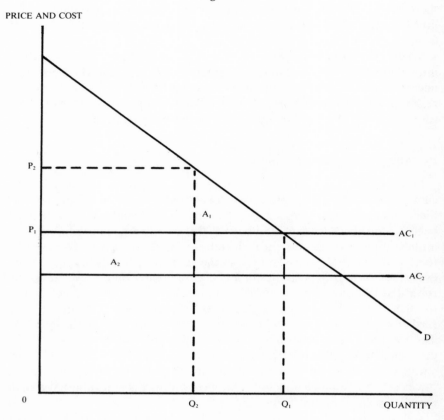

IV. PUBLIC POLICY TOWARD MERGERS

A. Judicial Treatment of Horizontal Mergers

In assessing the legality of a merger between two firms, the courts must decide whether the merger will result in a substantial lessening of competition or in a tendency to create a monopoly in any line of commerce in any section of the country. Thus, there is a need to define product and geographic markets. If the two firms are found to be competitors within the same product and geographic markets, the merger is horizontal. The next question is whether that particular merger substantially reduces competition. As we shall see, the judiciary has adopted an extremely hostile attitude toward horizontal mergers.

Product Market Definition. Defining the relevant product market is a surprisingly thorny problem in practice. Cross-elasticities of demand are very difficult to measure and, as a result, an analyst must rely upon price correlations and purchase patterns as a practical way of drawing inferences about the cross-elasticity of demand.[15] For the most part, however, the U.S. Supreme Court has not relied upon such evidence. In fact, the Court has adopted whatever product market definition was apt to lead to a government victory.

In its *Brown Shoe*[16] opinion, the Court recognized explicitly that the dimensions of a product market are drawn by the reasonable interchangeability of use or by the cross-elasticity of demand between the item in question and its potential substitutes. The Court ruled, however, that within a broad market there may also exist one or more well-defined submarkets, which can constitute a relevant line of commerce for antitrust purposes.[17] Critics of the submarket concept point out that serious errors can be committed when it is implemented in a particular case.[18] If a submarket is defined that omits products that curb the market power of the merging firms, then the analysis of competitive effect will be too severe. When one examines the cross-elasticity of demand and finds that a broad array of products are reasonably interchangeable, an analysis of competitive impact involving only a portion of that array will be misleading. No useful purpose is served by preventing unobjectionable mergers on the basis of faulty economic analysis.

The submarket concept has led to much mischief by the Court. Relying upon the *Brown Shoe* indicia, the Court in some instances has isolated some products from a broader group of products and treated the resulting submarket as economically relevant. This has resulted in the denial of what may have been innocent mergers. The abuse of the submarket concept was obvious in *Alcoa (Rome)*,[19] which involved Alcoa's acquisition of Rome Cable. Alcoa produced bare aluminum wire and cable and also insulated aluminum wire and cable. While bare aluminum conductor is a separate line of commerce, insulated conductor must compete with its copper counterpart. The Court, however, rejected this lower court finding of commercial reality and separated insulated copper and aluminum conductor into separate product markets. This approach makes gerrymandering of markets possible.

An even more egregious example of the Court's excesses is provided by the *Continental Can* case.[20] Continental Can, which made metal containers, acquired Hazel Atlas, which made glass jars. Although the lower court felt that metal and glass were separate products, the Supreme Court grouped them together because they competed in some uses. Discarding the niceties of reasonable interchangeability of use and cross-elasticity of demand, the Court ruled that the relevant line of commerce was metal and glass containers. The majority was not "concerned by the suggestion that if the product market is to be defined in these terms it must include plastic, paper, foil and any other materials competing for the same business." This lack of logic cannot be dismissed lightly. Given these precedents, it is clear that the Court can manipulate the product market definition to obtain any desired result in a merger case.

Geographic Market Definition. The economic tools that proved useful in defining the relevant product market are also useful in defining the relevant geographic market. Not surprisingly, however, the Court's treatment of geographic markets has been unsatisfactory. For example, in its *Pabst* decision,[21] the Court adopted a rather casual attitude toward geographic market definition. This case involved a merger between Pabst and Blatz, which the Antitrust Division challenged under Section 7. Using either the state of Wisconsin alone or the states of Illinois, Michigan, and Wisconsin as the relevant geographic market, the government claimed that the merger substantially lessened competition. The district court ruled in favor of Pabst because the government had failed to prove that either Wisconsin or the three-state area was a relevant geographic market. The U.S. Supreme Court reversed the lower court and expressed a lack of concern for carefully defining the market. According to the Court, Section 7 "requires merely that the Government prove the merger has substantial anticompetitive effect somewhere in the United States." Just how the government would go about proving this without defining a relevant geographic market was never made explicit.

The *Pabst* decision was rendered by the Warren Court in an era of extreme hostility toward mergers. Happily, a much different Court addressed the geographic market definition question in *Marine Bancorpor-*

ation,[22] which involved the merger of two banks in the State of Washington. The National Bank of Commerce (NBC) was located principally in Seattle and had no branch offices in Spokane. NBC wanted to acquire the Washington Trust Bank, which operated in Spokane. These banks did not compete with each other, and state banking laws precluded any practical way for NBC to enter the Spokane market except by acquiring one of the existing banks. The Court ruled against the government and recanted some of the unfortunate language in *Pabst.*

In its *Marine Bancorporation* decision, the Court tried to resurrect the requirement that a plaintiff establish a substantial anticompetitive effect within a sensibly defined geographic market. This effort resulted in an operationally empty pronouncement that a relevant geographic market is an area in which the "goods and services at issue are marketed to a significant degree by the acquired firm." Although its resurrection of the necessity for establishing a relevant market should be applauded, the Court provided little guidance on the sort of proof that will satisfy the requirement.

Establishing Anticompetitive Effect. At the U.S. Supreme Court, the standard for proving anticompetitive effect has revolved around market shares for many years. At least as early as the *Columbia Steel*[23] decision in 1948, market shares have been important. Following the Celler–Kefauver Amendment to Section 7 of the Clayton Act in 1950, however, the importance of market shares took a big leap forward.

In its *Brown Shoe* decision, the U.S. Supreme Court felt compelled to review the legislative history of the Celler–Kefauver amendment of Section 7. Among the factors that the Court described as being instrumental in the passage of the legislation was Congress's desire to provide the power to halt a merger trend. Moreover, according to the Court, Congress wanted to make it easier for the government to prevail by providing a lower standard of proof than the Sherman Act demanded. The Court noted that Congress did not propose any particular tests for defining the relevant markets, nor did it define the term *substantially.* Congress, however, did intend that a merger be viewed functionally in the context of the relevant industry. Finally, the Court noted that the language of Section 7 clearly indicates a concern with probabilities rather than with certainties.

Turning to the case at hand, the U.S. Supreme Court noted the product and geographic markets and then zeroed in on the market share of the merged firms, which is "one of the most important factors to be considered when determining the probable effects . . . on effective competition in the relevant market." The Court went on to find that a 5% share was important in a fragmented market. Moreover, a small share supposedly gained significance if a particular outlet was part of a strong national chain. Just what transformed a small share into something more significant remains a mystery.

The importance of market shares received a further boost in the following year when the Court decided the *Philadelphia National Bank* case.[24] The Philadelphia National Bank (PNB), second largest commercial bank in the Philadelphia area, merged with Girard Trust Corn Exchange Bank, third largest commercial bank of the 42 commercial banks in the four-county area around Philadelphia. The newly merged firm would have been the largest in the area with a market share of 34–36%.

In this case, the Court decided not to do any economic analysis. Noting a congressional concern with increases in concentration in the economy, the Court said that

[t]his intense congressional concern with the trend toward concentration warrants dispensing, in certain cases, with elaborate proof of market structure, market-behavior, or probable anticompetitive effects. Specifically, we think that a merger which produces a firm controlling an undue percentage share of the relevant market, and results in a significant increase in the concentration of firms in that market is so inherently likely to lessen competition substantially that it must be enjoined in the absence of evidence clearly showing that the merger is not likely to have such anticompetitive effects.

Incredibly, the Court felt that this "test is fully consonant with economic theory."

This cavalier attitude toward proof of adverse effect was not an isolated instance. In the *Continental Can* decision, the Court observed that "[w]here any merger is of such size as to be inherently suspect, elaborate proof of market structure, market behavior and probable anticompetitive effects may be dispensed with in view of Section 7's design to prevent undue concentration."

Summary. It is safe to say that before President Nixon began altering the character of the U.S. Supreme Court, a defendant in a merger case would not fare well. The Court gerrymandered product and geographic market definitions to put the merging parties in the worst light possible. Following that, the Court would use no economic analysis, but would find the requisite anticompetitive effect. This behavior was so pronounced that the late Justice Potter Stewart was moved to complain that "[t]he sole consistency that I can find is that in litigation under §7, the Government always wins."[25]

B. Department of Justice Attitude Toward Mergers

The attitude of the U.S. Department of Justice's Antitrust Division toward horizontal mergers is contained in its merger guidelines. In 1968, the Department of Justice published its first set of merger guidelines, which were designed to provide clear signals to the business community regarding the Antitrust Division's attitude toward mergers. These guidelines revealed a hostility toward horizontal mergers that paralleled that of the U.S. Supreme Court. By 1982, however, the Department of Justice was in the hands of people who were more sympathetic to the business community. The revised guidelines of 1982 reflected this change in attitude, as do the newest set of guidelines, which were published on June 14, 1984. The purpose of the guidelines continues to be to improve predictability of the Department's merger enforcement policy. Nonetheless, the Department will use the guidelines in conjunction with informed judgment regarding the factual setting and competitive conditions that surround the specific merger in question.

Horizontal Merger Standards. In examining horizontal mergers, the Department will use the Herfindahl–Hirschman Index (HHI), which it calculates by summing the squares of the individual market shares of all firms in the market. It ignores the decimal point in the calculation, so that if there were four firms with market shares of 10, 25, 30, and 35%, the HHI would be $(10)^2 + (25)^2 + (30)^2 + (35)^2 = 2850$. The Department divides the spectrum of market concentration as measured by the HHI into three regions that can be characterized broadly as unconcentrated (HHI below 1000), moderately concentrated (HHI between 1000 and 1800), and highly concentrated (HHI above 1800). An empirical study by the Department of the size dispersion of firms within markets indicates that the critical HHI thresholds at 1000 and 1800 correspond roughly to four-firm concentration ratios of 50% and 70%, respectively.

The general standards for horizontal mergers are as follows:

(a) *Post-merger HHI below 1000.* Markets in this region generally would be considered to be unconcentrated. Because implicit coordination among firms is likely to be difficult and because the prohibitions of Section 1 of the Sherman Act are usually an adequate response to any explicit collusion that might occur, the Department will not challenge mergers falling in this region, except in extraordinary circumstances.

(b) *Post-merger HHI between 1000 and 1800.* Because this region extends from the point at which the competitive concerns associated with concentration are raised to the point at which they become quite serious, generalization is particularly difficult. The Department, however, is unlikely to challenge a merger producing an increase in the HHI of less than 100 points. The Department is likely to challenge mergers in this region that produce an increase in the HHI of more than 100 points, unless the Department concludes that the merger is not likely substantially to lessen competition.

(c) *Post-merger HHI above 1800.*   Markets in this region generally are considered to be highly concentrated. Additional concentration resulting from mergers is a matter of significant competitive concern. The Department is unlikely, however, to challenge mergers producing an increase in the HHI of less than 50 points. The Department is likely to challenge mergers in this region that produce an increase in the HHI of more than 50 points, unless the Department concludes that the merger is not likely substantially to lessen competition.

Other Considerations.   The Department claims to have no interest in a mechanical approach to analyzing horizontal mergers. Thus, it will examine and consider other factors before making a final decision on whether to challenge a particular merger. These factors include changing market conditions, ease of entry, homogeneity of the product, special buyer characteristics, the ability of fringe firms to expand sales, the conduct of the firms in the market, and considerations of efficiency.

C.   Efficiency Considerations

Given the judicial attitude toward horizontal mergers and the U.S. Supreme Court's reluctance to engage in economic analysis, it would be rather surprising to find a careful examination of efficiency. The U.S. Department of Justice, however, would appear to be more receptive. The guidelines suggest that this is true.

Judicial Attitude Toward Efficiency.   No merger has ever been spared by the Court because it increased efficiency. In fact, the judiciary has been inexplicably hostile toward efficiency. For example, in *Brown Shoe*, the Court found that the merger of Brown Shoe and Kinney would lead to efficiencies that, in turn, would lead to lower prices. This, of course, would be competitively beneficial and, therefore, was not applauded by the Court. Instead, it was one of the reasons that the merger was condemned as the Court—protestations to the contrary notwithstanding—was concerned about competitors, not competition.

This economic illogic was not an isolated instance. In its *Bethlehem* decision,[26] the court pointed out that if a merger offends Section 7 in any relevant market, then "even demonstrable benefits are irrelevant and no defense." This theme was reiterated by Justice William O. Douglas in his *Clorox*[27] opinion: "Possible economies cannot be used as a defense to illegality. Congress was aware that some mergers which lessen competition may also result in economies, but it struck the balance in favor of protecting competition." As Bork (1978, p. 204) points out, the Court objected to Procter & Gamble's making Clorox more efficient.

Thus, the judicial system has not embraced an efficiency defense. On the contrary, the courts have considered efficiency to be irrelevant at best and actually offensive at worst.

Antitrust Division's Attitude Toward Efficiency. The Antitrust Division explicitly recognizes that many mergers are motivated by efficiency considerations. In many instances, mergers can increase the competitiveness of firms and result in price reductions for consumers. This recognition notwithstanding, the Antitrust Division does not consider efficiencies to be a defense to an otherwise anticompetitive merger. Instead, efficiency is just one of many factors that the Antitrust Division will consider in determining whether it should challenge a merger.[28]

In deciding whether to challenge a particular merger, the Antitrust Division recognizes the efficiency-enhancing potential of mergers generally. It is aware of the fact that mergers can increase the competitiveness of firms and thereby lead to price reductions for consumers. Both the guidelines and their accompanying statement, however, are silent on the situation described above in which a merger leads to both lower costs and higher prices.

If the merging firms establish by clear and convincing evidence that a merger will establish efficiencies, then the Antitrust Division may permit a merger that it would otherwise challenge. In this connection, the Antitrust Division recognizes that efficiencies may arise due to (1) achieving economies of scale; (2) better integration of production facilities; (3) plant specialization; (4) lower transportation costs; and (5) similar efficiencies relating to specific manufacturing, servicing, or distribution operations of the merging firms. In addition, the Antitrust Division is willing to consider efficiency claims resulting from reductions in general selling, administrative, and overhead expenses. It notes, however, that these are apt to be very difficult to demonstrate in practice. Finally, we should note that the Antitrust Division rejects claims of efficiencies if equivalent savings reasonably can be achieved by the parties through other means.

V. THE HEALTH CARE MARKET AND THE PERFORMANCE OF NONPROFIT ORGANIZATIONS

The nonprofit form of organization dominates the hospital industry. The reasons for this are not perfectly clear, but perhaps the most important motive is a belief that it is wrong to leave the provision of such a basic human need as health care to the dictates of the profit motive. In other words it may be "wrong" to make a profit from another human's suffering. Perhaps, also, it historically has been easier to raise capital for hospitals with the nonprofit organizational form. Possibly, too, there is a feeling that the profit sector would not provide enough resources for health care if left to its own devices. Finally, there may be distributive motives as well. Whatever the motive, it seems likely that the nonprofit form's dominance finds part of its roots, at least, in certain peculiarities of the health care industry that lead to what is widely regarded as market failure. This section first briefly sketches these market problems which are centered around information inadequacies and third-party reimbursement. Then, tax advantages and other discriminatory benefits afforded to the nonprofits are examined. Next, efficiency and cost shortcomings of nonprofits, even in the presence of their preferential treatment, are explored. Finally, it is determined that these deficiencies are caused, at least in part, by managerial slack brought about by the incentives of nonprofit managers, which are different from those of their for-profit counterparts, and also by the lack of competitive check because the for-profits do not enjoy the same advantages.

A. The Health Care Market

The special problems of the health care industry are well known (Frech, 1984; Clark, 1980 provide good summaries) and need not be given lengthy treatment here. These problems revolve around uncertainty and the lack of market information (Arrow, 1963). More specifically, in a modern society with very extensive medical knowledge and with complex technologies available for treatment, consumers are necessarily ignorant of the requisite knowledge for informed market choice. They can't possibly have sufficient knowledge of symptoms, causes, diagnosis, and treatments to evaluate the adequacy of the care provided by their physicians and hospitals. To be sure, the medical profession is ethically bound to provide these services in such a way that the physician must put the needs of the patient first. But even granting this ethical approach by physicians, the lack of information makes informed choice by consumers very difficult. If consumers are unable to evaluate the quality of the care they receive, then they are not capable of making good choices among competing products based on price. If consumers cannot make choices based on price because of this information problem, viable price competition is difficult to achieve.

The effect of consumer ignorance on competition in health care is aggravated by the dominance of third-party payment for health expenditures (Frech, 1984, p. 3). Third-party payments reduce the incentives for consumers to search for the best price available in the market. If insurers will pay all or a large percentage of his health care bill, there is no reward to the consumer for seeking out a lower price, even if he has the necessary information to do so. It might seem that insurers would take on the role of evaluating sophisticated medical procedures in the face of the consumer's inability to do so. "But the insurer faces another kind of information problem: the sheer cost of gathering full information about the history and symptoms of a particular patient, and applying to it in an objective fashion an articulated, agreed-upon set of medical principles concerning diagnosis, prognosis, and treatment. To the extent that the insurer defers to the physician's 'discretion' and 'judgment,' he foregoes the role of monitor" (Clark, 1980, p. 1421). The task of evaluating physicians' judgment would be monumental and aggravated by the fact that competent medical personnel may disagree about the merits of different treatments.

If consumers and insurers have a problem with information, then so too does society:

> The possible inadequacy of prevailing medical approaches is suggested by evidence that the great increase over the last twenty years in the proportion of the gross national product devoted to health care has had little impact on the health status of the American population. Medical experts, journalists, and other commentators have focused on portions of the problem, such as the tenuous relationship between long hospital stays and successful recovery from certain medical problems. But society as a whole, when allocating resources to or consuming health care, manifests an almost childlike faith that modern medicine and the practices conventionally associated with it are rational in cost-benefit terms. Many doctors do know better and try to convey to their patients some sense of the limits of medicine. But the full seriousness of the problem seems to be appreciated by only a small core of public policy analysts.[29]

If consumers and insurers have inadequate information for rational market choice, if indeed even medical experts disagree on the cost-effectiveness of treatments, the implications for meaningful competition in the market for health care are serious.

B. The Nonprofit Hospitals and Their Performance

The nonprofit hospitals may well enjoy exemption from Section 7 of the Clayton Act. If mergers of nonprofit hospitals are permitted, while those of for-profit hospitals are not, there are serious implications for efficiency in the hospital industry where the nonprofit hospitals dominate. These implications may be all the more serious because of the tax and operating advantages that the nonprofits enjoy. This follows because the special cost advantages enjoyed by the nonprofit hospitals may very well be dissipated "because" of their organizational form.

Professor Robert Clark has documented the disparate treatment accorded the nonprofits, pointing out that "numerous statutes, regulations, and judicial doctrines discriminate against for-profit hospitals." State and local governments exempt nonprofit hospitals from property taxes. Gifts to nonprofit hospitals are deductible from federal income taxes, while those to for-profits are not. Nonprofits are taxed only for the amount of actual unemployment claims filed, while for-profit hospitals are taxed according to payroll, usually a higher amount. Federal grants for the development of health maintenance organizations (HMOs) are provided to for-profit hospitals only if they are to be located in an area that is medically underserved. The same applies to loans. Medicare reimbursements call for "necessary and proper" costs of rendering services, included in which is a fair return on equity. But this has not been interpreted to include income taxes, resulting in a lower rate of return when adjusted for taxes. Clark goes on to list a host of other ways in which federal policies discriminate against the for-profits.

Tax and other discriminatory policies, then, afford the nonprofits considerable competitive advantage. In addition to this advantage, Clark found the for-profits to be dramatically smaller. This would mean that cost savings resulting from any economies of scale that exist—and most would grant that they do exist—would fall to the nonprofits also. If nonprofits have cost advantages because of favorable treatment and also because of economies of scale, then one would expect, of course, that they would provide services at lower cost than would their for-profit competitors. But just the opposite is true. In spite of lower occupancy rates, the for-profits experienced lower costs. This seems to be attributed to shorter lengths of stay in for-profits for similar procedures and also, in part, to their smaller amounts of cost-generating resources. If nonprofits have these cost advantages and still have higher costs, then one would think that they must be providing higher-quality services because of greater concern for patients and a reduced concern for profits. But this is not true either. The evidence that exists shows no quality difference between nonprofits and for-profits.

If nonprofits enjoy this cost advantage and also provide a similar quality of service while still experiencing higher costs than for-profits, then they must be less efficient. The reasons for this, of course, lie in the very nature of their nonprofit status and the incentives that that status implies.

Kenneth Clarkson (1972) finds that differences in incentives and, therefore, differences in efficiencies between nonprofits and for-profits have their roots in the differences in property rights invested in owners and managers. Owners or trustees of for-profits have exclusive rights to pecuniary and nonpecuniary benefits that derive from the production of hospital services. They impose rules and regulations on their managers that are designed to maximize those benefits. Indeed, managers are often afforded partial ownership rights to insure that they, insofar as possible, share the same goals as the owners. Increased profits and increased capital values, then, bring rewards to the managers and provide them with a direct stake in the efficiency with which services are provided.

In contrast, the trustees of nonproprietary hospitals do not have exclusive rights to these same pecuniary and nonpecuniary benefits. Nor can they assign these rights to managers, providing them with incentives to maximize the firm's wealth. Nonprofit managers, then, find a much reduced link between their own welfare and the wealth of the firm. Consequently, their interest in enhancing the efficiency of the firm is much less than that of the for-profit manager and, predictably, managerial slack is much greater. This managerial slack, attributable to the different incentives faced by the nonprofit manager, finds expression in many ways: less rigorous supervision of employees to the degree that close supervision, or say night-shift supervision, is unpleasant; hiring practices that tend to rely on credentials such as academic degrees rather than on harder-to-obtain indications of performance ability; much greater variance in input selection among non-profits, indicating that input selection is not as much constrained by market forces as it is with the for-profits; less vigorous collection of bad debts, indicating less pressure to increase revenues; and the belief by suppliers that nonprofit managers are less price-conscious in their purchasing efforts.[30]

In short, cost advantages enjoyed by the nonprofits, advantages which might very well be extracted by for-profits in the form of current income and increased value of the firm, may be dissipated to a large degree by managerial slack which lessens efficiency and increases cost. The ability to survive these inefficiencies, while largely attributable to third-party payments and the information problems with health care noted above, may also in part lie in the lack of competitive check by the for-profits which are not partner to those same advantages.

VI. CONCLUSIONS

We have noted above that the motives for horizontal merger include the attainment of market power, the achievement of economic efficiencies, or both. We have also noted that due to ambiguities in the statutes it is possible that nonprofits enjoy exemption from the merger provisions of Clayton 7 while the for-profits do not. While not taking a position as to what the overall policy posture should be toward mergers in the hospital industry, we do argue here that disparate treatment of nonprofits and for-profits can only have negative effects on economic efficiency. Further, the favorable treatment accorded the nonprofits under tax and other discriminatory policies makes it even more compelling that for-profits and nonprofits be afforded equal merger treatment. This is because the favorable treatment that the nonprofits receive gives them cost advantages that they apparently dissipate, at least in part. This, in turn, is because the incentives of nonprofit managers, as opposed to those of for-profit managers, do not dispose them to operate in an efficiency-enhancing way. The removal of a competitive check on their behavior by allowing favorable merger treatment, thus placing the for-profits at further disadvantage, would only serve to aggravate this situation. Since the nonprofit form dominates the hospital industry, anything that tends to decrease their efficiency is a serious matter.

In Section III it was pointed out that mergers that increase market power without any increase in efficiency are unambiguously bad since they raise price, reduce output, and result in a corresponding decrease in consumer welfare. If mergers of this type have unambiguously negative results, it makes no sense to permit them for nonprofits or for-profits.

But some mergers are undertaken in a quest for higher profits by reducing costs, usually through the achievement of economies of scale. These mergers lead to excess profits in the short run, but if no barriers to entry are erected,[31] these profits will encourage new firms to enter driving profits back down to the competitive level. The results of this kind of merger are unambiguously positive, and they should be permitted for the for-profit hospitals as well as for the nonprofit hospitals. If only nonprofits are permitted to pursue this type of merger, however, new entrants would not be attracted and the nonprofits would be left with an additional cost advantage over their for-profit counterparts. Disparate treatment in this situation is wrong for two reasons: first, it denies the cost efficiencies to the for-profits, thereby causing more resources to be devoted to health care than are necessary; and second, it protects the nonprofits from for-profit competition, permitting them to dissipate their gains in the ways discussed in the preceding section. Clearly, preferential treatment for nonprofits in the area of efficiency enhancing mergers has negative results for society.

Finally, there are those mergers that result in market power and also enhance efficiency through cost reductions. In Section III it was noted that if consumer welfare is the goal of merger policy, then policymakers must weigh the negative effects associated with increased market power (i.e., the deadweight loss associated with reduced output) against the positive effects (the lower average cost of producing the reduced quantity). Here, too, there is no reason for disparate treatment. If there are net benefits to consumers, then mergers should be allowed for both for-profits and nonprofits. If nonprofits are permitted to merge while for-profits are not, then consumer welfare will be reduced. First, to the degree that there are net efficiency gains from a merger and if that merger is forbidden for a for-profit hospital, consumer welfare will be less than it would be otherwise. Second, once again, if nonprofits are permitted to merge and for-profits are not, then it is likely that the nonprofits will dissipate at least part of their efficiency gains because of the absence of a competitive check.

In sum, while it is beyond the scope of this paper to examine the question of what overall merger policy should be toward the hospital industry, it seems clear from the standpoint of efficiency that disparate treatment can only do harm. If nonprofits are indeed exempt from the provisions of Clayton 7, then this is not good and public policy should be reexamined. In an industry where cost containment is a major problem, a policy which needlessly promotes inefficiency and puts upward pressure on costs is clearly wrong.

ACKNOWLEDGMENTS

The authors appreciate the financial support provided by the Public Policy Research Center at the University of Florida and a grant from the University of Tampa.

NOTES

1. While not all commentators agree that the sole purpose of the antitrust laws is to promote economic efficiency and while many would argue that they were designed instead to serve a broader range of political and social goals, most would agree that economic efficiency is an important, if not the primary, goal. For a summary of different opinions on the goals of antitrust see Blair and Fesmire (1986).

2. For an excellent historical account of the Sherman Act, see Thorelli (1954). Another historical account that includes an examination of the early enforcement is provided by Letwin (1965).

3. The current reform proposals of the Reagan administration demand that something stronger than a mere possibility be shown.

4. This was pointed out by Miles (1984, pp.260–262) and by Singer (1985, pp.6–7).

5. For a provocative discussion, see Stigler (1950).

6. For some empirical evidence, see Hay and Kelley (1974) and Fraas and Greer (1977). The theory is set out in Scherer (1980) and Blair and Kaserman (1985).

7. The seminal contribution is provided by Chamberlin (1933). For a modern treatment of tacit collusion that casts some doubt on its sensibility, see Spence (1978). For an analysis of the antitrust enforcement problems, see chap. 8 in Blair and Kaserman (1985).

8. Williamson (1968) provided the first formal analysis of the welfare trade-offs associated with efficiency enhancing mergers. Bork (1978) used Williamson's model in his devastating critique of current merger policy.

9. If average cost is constant, then marginal cost, the amount that is added to total cost when an additional unit is produced, must also be constant and equal to average cost. If marginal cost were greater than average cost, then an extra unit of production would add more to total cost than the previous average and the average would rise. If marginal cost were less than the previous average, then the extra unit would cause average cost to fall. See Blair and Kenny (1982, pp.91–94, 104).

10. Price equal to average cost results in zero economic profit. Zero economic profit, however, means that the firm is earning a normal profit. Economists, interested in resource allocation, include in total cost all payments required to attract and hold resources for the firm. A normal profit is required to keep the entrepreneur, an important resource, in the

business. When price is equal to average cost, then firms are earning what is called a competitive return or a normal profit. See Blair and Kenny (1982, pp.118–120, 376–379).

11. Competitive firms are restricted in their ability to increase price by the existence of many rivals. A merger, because it eliminates competitors to whom a firm's customers might switch, may give the firm the ability to raise price with a smaller loss of sales than would be the case in a more competitive atmosphere.

12. Area A_1 is often called a "deadweight loss." This is because those resources freed by the cutback in monopoly output will find their way into the production of other goods. If it is assumed that these other goods are produced in competitive industries, then price (the value consumers place on the goods) will equal marginal cost MC. In contrast, the output that is sacrificed by the monopoly has a value (P) greater than MC. The difference in the price of the new goods to be produced in presumably competitive industries and the price of the goods sacrificed by the monopoly represents the value lost to society, the "deadweight loss." See Hotelling (1938) and Willig (1976) for extended discussions.

13. These cost reductions measure the amount of resources that are freed by the efficiency gains, resources that can be used to produce other goods that will benefit society and thus increase its welfare. In contrast to the deadweight loss measured by area A_1, area A_2 represents a real saving of resources for society. These resources are free to produce additional goods in other, presumably competitive industries. The fact that these savings also represent increased profits for the producer is thought to be of no significance. Posner (1975), however, argues that these monopoly profits provide an incentive for firms to expend resources in the socially unproductive pursuit of monopoly status.

14. Fox (1981), however, argues that even if you accept the idea that efficiency is the goal of antitrust, the policy problem is not resolved because there are alternative means to the efficiency ends. She cites three different means of enhancing efficiency. One approach is for antitrust authorities to challenge only behavior that tends to decrease output. But even behavior that restricts output should not always be prevented if there are cost savings involved, as we have seen above. The second approach is to promote business autonomy. Business firms strive to maximize profits, which requires that firms minimize their costs. Since firms know best how to minimize their costs, the best way to maximize efficiency in the economy is to give firms the freedom to do what they want. The third approach is to preserve competition as a process. This approach centers on an environment that is conducive to vigorous rivalry and, therefore, to efficiency. While proponents of all approaches share the value of an environment conducive to rivalry, those who stress preserving competition as a process reject business autonomy as the proper means to this end and also reject output limitation as an exclusive guide to policy.

15. See Blair and Kaserman (1985, pp.106–110) for a discussion of this approach to defining the relevant product market.

16. *Brown Shoe Company, Inc.* v. *United States*, 370 U.S. 294 (1962).

17. The Court found that "[t]he boundaries of such a submarket may be determined by examining such practical indicia as (1) industry or public recognition of the submarket as a separate economic entity, (2) the product's peculiar characteristics and uses, (3) unique production facilities, (4) distinct customers, (5) distinct prices, (6) sensitivity to price changes, and (7) specialized vendors."

18. A stunning critique is provided by Maisel (1983).

19. *United States* v. *Aluminum Company of America (Rome Cable)*, 377 U.S. 271 (1964).

20. *United States* v. *Continental Can Company*, 378 U.S. 441 (1964).

21. *United States* v. *Pabst Brewing Company*, 384 U.S. 546 (1966).

22. *United States* v. *Marine Bancorporation, Inc.*, 418 U.S. 602 (1974).

23. *United States* v. *Columbia Steel Company*, 334 U.S. 495 (1948).

24. *United States* v. *Philadelphia National Bank*, 374 U.S. 321 (1963).

25. *United States* v. *Von's Grocery Company*, 384 U.S. 270 (1966), Justice Stewart's dissenting opinion.

26. *United States* v. *Bethlehem Steel Corp.*, 168 F. Supp. 576 (S.D.N.Y. 1958).

27. *Federal Trade Commission* v. *Procter & Gamble Co.*, 386 U.S. 568, 580 (1967).

28. The Antitrust Division's official attitude toward efficiency is contained in its latest merger guidelines (Guidelines, 1984 §3.5) and the statement that accompanied their release.

29. Much of the remainder of this section draws heavily on Clark (1980). His interesting article examines the evidence for the alternative hypotheses that nonprofit hospitals serve consumers as either fiduciaries or exploiters. He concludes that the evidence does not support the idea that nonprofit hospitals act as fiduciaries and argues that the legal treatment accorded for-profit and nonprofit hospitals should be equal.

30. This managerial slack seems similar in some respects to Leibenstein's X-inefficiency. Leibenstein suggested that efficiency losses may stem from nonmaximizing behavior. He felt that neither individuals nor firms work as hard, nor do they search for information as effectively as they could. This emphasis on motivation is important since the relationship between inputs and outputs is not determinant because (1) contracts for labor are not complete, which makes monitoring very important; (2) not all factors of production are marketed or available on the same terms to all buyers (e.g., managerial inputs may not be available and if available, tend to be heterogeneous); (3) the production function is not completely specified nor known; and (4) interdependence and uncertainty lead competing firms to cooperate tacitly with each other in some respects and to imitate each other with respect to technique to some degree. That is, Leibenstein said firms do not minimize costs (Leibenstein, 1966; Shelton, 1967). For a summary of X-inefficiency, see Blair and Kaserman (1985).

While similar in effect, Clark's managerial slack finds its source not in monopoly power, but in the property rights and differing incentives of nonprofit managers.

31. It is clear that some very substantial barriers to entry exist in the form of certificates of need. Nonetheless, the existence of this type of barrier to efficiency gains, if it exists, does not negate the thesis that disparate treatment makes little sense.

REFERENCES

Albertson, James B. (1985), "Hospital Antitrust: The Merging Hospital and the Resulting Exposure to Antitrust Merger and Monopolization Laws." *Washburn Law Journal* 24(2):300–326.

Arrow, Kenneth (1963), "Uncertainty and the Welfare Economics of Medical Care." *American Economic Review* 53(4):941–973.

Blackstone, Erwin A. and Joseph P. Fuhr, Jr. (1985), "Hospital Mergers and Antitrust: An Economic Analysis." Unpublished paper presented at American Economic Association meetings, December 28, 1985.

Blair, Roger D. and David L. Kaserman (1985), *Antitrust Economics.* Homewood, IL: Irwin.

Blair, Roger D. and Lawrence W. Kenny (1982), *Microeconomics For Managerial Decision Making.* New York: McGraw-Hill.

Blair, Roger D. and James M. Fesmire (1986), "Maximum Price Fixing and the Goals of Antitrust." *Syracuse Law Review* 37(1):43–77.

Bork, Robert H. (1978), *The Antitrust Paradox.* New York: Basic Books.

Chamberlin, E.H. (1933), *The Theory of Monopolistic Competition.* Cambridge, MA: Harvard University Press.

Clark, Robert Charles (1980), "Does the Nonprofit Form Fit the Hospital Industry." *Harvard Law Review* 93(5):1416–1489.

Clarkson, Kenneth W. (1972), "Some Implications of Property Rights in Hospital Management." *Journal of Law and Economics* 15(2):363–384.

Davis, Karen (1971), "Economic Theories of Behavior in Nonprofit, Private Hospitals." *Economic and Business Bulletin* 24(1):1–13.
Ellman, Ira Mark (1982), "Another Theory of Nonprofit Corporations." *Michigan Law Review* 93(5):1416–1489.
Fox, Eleanor (1981), "The Modernization of Antitrust: A New Equilibrium." *Cornell Law Review* 66(5):1140–1192.
Fraas, Arthur G. and Douglas F. Greer (1977), "Market Structure and Price Collusion: An Empirical Analysis." *Journal of Industrial Economics* 26(1):29–33.
Frech, H.E. (1984), "Competition in Medical Care: Research and Policy." In R.M. Scheffler and L.R. Rossiter (Eds.), *Advances in Health Economics and Health Services Research*, Vol V. Greenwich, CT: JAI Press, pp. 1–27.
Ginsburg, Douglas H. (1986), "Remarks to NHLA on Health Care and Antitrust Reform Legislation." Reproduced in *Antitrust & Trade Regulation Report* 50(4):174–176.
Hay, George A. and Daniel Kelley (1974), "An Empirical Survey of Price Fixing Conspiracies." *Journal of Law and Economics* 17(1):13–38.
Hotelling, Harold (1938), "The General Welfare in Relation to Problems of Taxation and of Railway and Utility Rates." *Econometrica* 6(3):242–269.
Leibenstein, Harvey (1966), "Allocative Efficing v. X-inefficiency." *American Economic Review* 56(3):392–415.
Letwin, William (1965), *Law and Economic Policy in America*. New York: Random House.
Maisel, Lawrence E. (1983), "Submarkets in Merger and Monopolization Cases." *Georgetown Law Journal* 72(1):39–71.
Miles, John J. (1984), "Hospital Mergers and the Antitrust Laws: An Overview." *Antitrust Bulletin XXIX* (2):253–299.
Posner, Richard (1975), "The Social Costs of Monopoly and Regulation." *Journal of Political Economy* 83(4):807–828.
Scherer, F.M. (1980), *Industrial Market Structure and Economic Performance*. Boston: Houghton Mifflin.
Schramm, Carl J. and Steven C. Renn (1984), "Hospital Mergers, Market Concentration and the Herfindahl-Hirschman Index." *Emory Law Journal* 33(4):869–888.
Senate Report No. 698, to accompany H.R. 15,657, 63d Congress, 2d session (1914).
Shelton, John P. (1967) "Allocative Efficiency v. X-inefficiency: Comment," *American Economic Review* 57(5):1252–1258.
Singer, Toby G. (1985), "Application of Federal Antitrust Law to Mergers of Competing Hospitals." Materials accompanying remarks presented at the 19th New England Antitrust Conference, November 8.
Spence, Michael (1978), "Tacit Co-ordination and Imperfect Information." *Canadian Journal of Economics* 11(3):490–505.
Stigler, George J. (1950), "Monopoly and Oligopoly by Merger." *American Economic Review* 40(2):23–34.
Thorelli, Hans B. (1954), *The Federal Antitrust Policy*. Reading, MA: Allen & Unwin.
United States Department of Justice Merger Guidelines, reprinted in *Antitrust & Trade Regulation Report* (June 14, 1984).
Williamson, Oliver E. (1968), "Economies as an Antitrust Defense: The Welfare Tradeoffs." *American Economic Review* 58(1):18–34.
Willig, Robert (1976), "Consumer's Surplus Without Apology." *American Economic Review* 66(4):589–597.

ANTITRUST CONSIDERATIONS FOR HOSPITAL MERGERS:

MARKET DEFINITION AND MARKET CONCENTRATION

Ronald P. Wilder and Philip Jacobs

I. INTRODUCTION

As the importance of privately owned hospitals in the United States increases, and as new institutional arrangements for the provision of health
care services proliferate, it is reasonable to expect an increase in the in-
cidence of hospital mergers. Because hospital markets tend to be local or
regional in scope, and because hospitals differ with respect to the array of
services offered, hospital mergers may or not involve anticompetitive effects. The purpose of this paper is to analyze the likely anticompetitive
effects of hospital mergers, considering both geographic market definition
and product market definition in analyzing alternative merger scenarios.

Both geographic market and product market definitions for hospitals are
based on the interchangeability or cross-price elasticity of the services
offered, as viewed by the consumers. Two hospitals are in the same geographic market if consumers (or their physician agents) consider them to
be reasonably interchangeable when making the decision regarding where
to seek care. Two hospitals are in the same product market if consumers

Advances in Health Economics and Health Services Research, Vol. 7, pgs. 245–262.
Copyright © 1987 by JAI Press Inc.
ISBN: 0-89232-573-9

consider their offerings of a particular service to be reasonably interchangeable.

The analysis will consider hospital concentration in local and regional markets as measured by the Herfindahl Index. Empirical estimates of hospital concentration for various procedures and services in South Carolina will be presented. These concentration data will be considered in the light of the U.S. Department of Justice merger guidelines of 1982 and 1984. In contrast to most of the previous discussion of hospital markets and market concentration, we develop the argument that the individual diagnosis or procedure, rather than the general cluster of hospital services as a whole, is the relevant product market.

II. HOSPITAL MARKET STRUCTURES: CAUSES AND EFFECTS

A. Hospital Concentration: Causes

Concentration in hospital markets is generally discussed as if hospital service markets were highly localized. Thus Luft (1984/85) refers to 5-and 15-mile distances between hospitals as two alternative measures of potential linkages from a competitive standpoint. Farley (1985) uses the county as the market measure, while Joskow (1980) uses the Standard Metropolitan Statistical Area (SMSA). Both Farley and Joskow imply that counties or non-SMSA cities with a single hospital are monopolistic markets (i.e., have a value for the Herfindahl ratio of 1). If this is the case then much of the hospital industry is very highly concentrated, since so many towns and counties have only one or two hospitals.

What are the potential causes of concentration in the hospital industry? First, there is the frequently cited factor of economies of scale relative to market size. In fact, there seems to be some question about the existence of scale economies in hospitals (Lave and Lave, 1984). To the extent that scale economies do exist, there is some question as to whether they would have had a major impact on concentration. Suppliers gain market share advantages from scale economies when they can take advantage of their lower costs by pricing below levels set by smaller, higher-cost competitors. Until recently, consumers in the hospital industry have been blind to cost differentials among producers because of relatively complete insurance coverage for hospital care. As a result, suppliers would not have been able to take advantage of cost differentials in order to enlarge their market shares. The hospital industry is now entering a new phase where a new set of economies (those associated with multiplant firms) and more price conscious purchasers [employers, third-party insurers, and health maintenance organizations (HMOs)] may lead to increased price competition and perhaps more concentrated market shares.

A second potential factor influencing concentration is patient transportation costs. If these costs impose a heavy burden on patients, then the potential market is narrowed. On the other hand, considerable patient mobility will reduce concentration by widening the market.

A third cause of concentration is related to the quality factor which is associated with a negative relationship between postoperative mortality (or just unsuccessful outcomes) and the scale of operations for certain complex surgical procedures (Luft, Bunker, and Enthoven, 1979). Hospitals which perform these procedures on a small scale will have high expected mortality rates; that is, high expected mortality costs will be imposed on patients. Unlike hospital operating costs, patients cannot be shielded from expected mortality costs. They can reduce these costs, however, by going to medical centers where scale of operations are higher. The reduction in the number of hospitals performing these procedures does not automatically translate into higher concentration ratios. If patients are willing to incur increased travel costs to reduce expected mortality costs, the market becomes wider and several widely dispersed major medical centers may serve a given area. It should be pointed out that this analysis requires examining separate markets for different diagnoses, viewing the hospital as a multi-product firm (Goldfarb, Hornbrook, and Rafferty, 1980).

Fourth, mergers will lead to increased concentration, as long as the mergers occur in the relevant market areas. In recent years a "multihospital" movement has been identified as a growing phenomenon. (Mason, 1979). This movement has resulted from takeovers and mergers of both nonprofit and for-profit corporate entities.

Finally, regulation has had an effect on hospital concentration. Salkever and Bice (1976) have shown that hospital capital investment review regulation has hampered hospital bed expansion and presumably the *number* of competing entities in a given market.

B. Hospital Concentration: Effects

Competition among hospitals can have several effects. First, it potentially can influence hospital prices. It has traditionally been thought that this effect is minimal because of the widespread existence of hospitalization insurance. Because patient out-of-pocket payments are so low in this sector, patients have not been sensitive to price differentials between hospitals (Joskow, 1980). However, this view is changing because of the growing role of corporations and third-party insurers as interested buyers. Phenomena such as preferred provider organizations and Medicaid contract bidding (Christianson, 1984) are creating potential volume increases in response to hospital pricing decisions. As a result, increased price competition and concentration may be taking on a new role of importance.

The "traditional" view of hospital competition is that such competition is of the nonprice variety (Joskow, 1980; Farley, 1985). Physicians have dual roles as agents of their patients as well as "customers" of hospitals. Hospitals can bid for physicians' business by offering them a wider scope of services and excess capacity in these services. In the process of doing so, of course, hospitals' costs are raised; but since price competition has not been a major factor in this industry, it has not generally been a constraining element. In those situations where price competition plays a growing role, hospital budgets will be more constrained and such growth in the scope and capacity of services may be curtailed.

III. CONCEPTUAL ISSUES IN MARKET DEFINITION: THE CASE OF HOSPITAL MARKETS

The plane of competition in economic analysis is the market. A market is a group of competing sellers and competing buyers who enter into exchange transactions relating to a particular good or service. The market has two dimensions: the product dimension and the geographic or spatial dimension. The product dimension of markets is related to the interchangeability in use of a group of similar commodities. The geographic or spatial dimension considers the market boundaries related to the location of buyers and sellers. Because of transportation costs, groups of buyers and sellers of the same products may be in different markets due to location. This section considers market definition for horizontal mergers with respect to both of these market dimensions.

A. The Relevant Product Market or Markets

In its decision in the du Pont cellophane case, the U.S. Supreme Court stated that the market is made up of "products that have reasonable interchangeability for the purposes for which they are produced—price, use and qualities considered." This decision appears to embody the economist's concept of cross-price elasticity of demand, which is based on the responsiveness of the quantity demanded for one supplier to the price changes of a competing supplier. If cross-price elasticity of demand is relatively high, the two suppliers are in the same product market; if relatively low, they are in separate product markets.

The price of hospital services is a more complex concept than is the price of other consumer goods and services. The presence of third-party payers means that individuals frequently experience a marginal out of pocket cost which is zero or near zero, even when a medical procedure requiring a large expenditure of resources is received by the individual. Does this feature of hospital care prices mean that the cross-price elasticity concept is not relevant for hospital markets? We believe that the concept is still relevant, but that its application requires some care and additional analysis.

The price of hospital services to the patient includes the following components:

1. The out-of-pocket cost of care to the patient, which may be quite different from the resource cost, due to third-party payments
2. The travel and time costs to the patient and to family members
3. The expected or probability costs associated with the risk of disability or death for the particular procedure

Even if the out-of-pocket cost to the patient is low, the other cost components may be of great importance, so that competition among hospitals affects the choices of patients and physicians. Our discussion of cross-price elasticity of demand in this paper is framed in the context of this concept of price, and its applicability to hospital markets is maintained even when out-of-pocket cost is low or zero.

This concept is the foundation for product market definition, but is not the whole story. First, the cross-price elasticity of demand is likely to vary with the level of price, so that some suppliers that are not reasonably close substitutes at low prices may be substitutes at higher prices. Similarly, firms that are not producing for a particular market at relatively low prices may begin production at a sufficiently high price. In the case of hospitals, for example, the growth of outpatient surgical centers as a substitute for in-patient surgery can be viewed as a market response to the relatively high per diem cost of hospitalization. Hospitals may also expand existing product lines or add new product lines in response to price changes. The elasticity of supply related to such responses is limited, however, by the existence of procedure-specific capital equipment and physician specialization.

Because market definition is crucial to the determination of market shares of firms participating in a merger, the Justice Department's merger guidelines have devoted explicit attention to this issue. The 1968 merger guidelines, for example, stated that

[a] market is any grouping of sales . . . in which each of the firms whose sales are included enjoys some advantage in competing with those firms whose sales are not included. . . . The sales of any product or service which is distinguishable as a matter of commercial practice from other products or services will ordinarily constitute a relevant product market, even though, from the standpoint of most purchasers, other products may be reasonably, but not perfectly, interchangeable with it in terms of price, quality and use . . . " (quoted by Posner, 1976, pp. 130-131).

As Posner suggests, this approach to product market definition is very strict, almost suggesting that only perfect substitutes are included in the same product market. This approach would tend to produce high market shares and to increase the likelihood that a merger would be challenged. The approach of the 1968 guidelines is thus consistent with the enforcement tradition of the 1950s and 1960s of taking a very strict position on horizontal mergers.

The 1982 and 1984 merger guidelines take a position which is also closely related to the cross-price elasticity concept:

> In general, the Department will include in the product market a group of products such that a hypothetical firm that was the only present and future seller of those products ["monopolist"] could profitably impose a "small but significant and non-transitory" increase in price. . . . The Department generally will consider the relevant product market to be the smallest group of products that satisfies this test (1984 Merger Guidelines, pp. 33–34).

This version of the merger guidelines applies a more conceptually rigorous statement of product substitution and conforms more closely to the economist's concept of cross-elasticity of demand than did the 1968 guidelines. In general this approach to product market definition could be expected to be associated with a more lenient approach to horizontal mergers, which appears to have been the general approach of the Reagan administration's Justice Department.

In applying these market definition concepts to hospital markets, we take the position that the relevant product market for hospital mergers is the diagnosis group or the medical procedure, rather than the cluster of hospital services as a whole. The basis for this position is, once again, the economic concept of cross-elasticity of demand. We would expect the cross-price elasticity of demand between appendectomies and normal labor and delivery to be zero from the point of view of the patient or the patient's physician-agent. The patient does not select from a menu of diagnoses based on price. The patient, on the other hand, may switch among hospitals or between a hospital and a nonhospital mode of service delivery for a particular diagnosis on the basis of price.

This approach to market definition for hospitals could produce higher or lower market shares than an approach based on hospital services as a general product line. Not all hospitals produce all medical procedures, especially those procedures which involve very high fixed costs and specialized staffs, such as cardiovascular surgery. The markets for such procedures would be more highly concentrated under the market definition approach taken here than under an approach which considers hospital services in general as the relevant product market. For medical procedures which may be performed on an inpatient hospital basis, on a hospital outpatient basis, or in nonhospital outpatient clinics, the relevant product market should include all of these alternative delivery modes. (Increasingly, in many cases the relevant product market will include different procedures for the same diagnoses, e.g., surgery or medical management for tonsillitis or pyloric stenosis.) In product markets such as these, our approach to market definition would produce lower market shares than a more general hospital service approach.

Horizontal mergers are likely to become increasingly popular in hospital markets as investor-owned hospital chains seek to expand their activities and as publicly owned hospitals begin to engage in mergers as a defensive measure. Certificate-of-need regulation makes merger in hospital markets an even more attractive means of entry or market extension than it would be in other sectors of the economy. All of three recent challenged mergers in hospital markets involved for-profit hospital chains: (*AMI,* FTC docket No. 9158; *American Medicorp* v. *Humana, Inc.,* 445 F. Supp. 589, 605 (E.D. Pa. 1977)—both cases cited in Alpert and McCarthy (1985). The October 1985 Federal Trade Commission (FTC) decision of the Hospital Corporation of America (HCA) acquisition of Hospital Affiliates International (HAI) is the most recent antitrust judgment regarding hospitals. Because of its importance, it will be considered at greater length below (*Hospital Corp. of America,* CCH Trade Regulation Reports, para. 22,301, 1985).

B. The Relevant Geographic Market

In addition to the product market dimension of markets, the geographic or spatial dimension is also an important element of market definition. For most goods and services, buyers and sellers are located at fixed points. Engaging in exchange then imposes transportation costs on buyers, sellers, or both. Because hospital services are traditionally delivered at the premises of the hospital, most of the transportation costs in hospital services are borne by the buyer, who must travel to the site of the selected hospital. The transportation costs include not only the out-of-pocket costs of travel, but also the time costs associated with travel, including the time costs of spouses or other close relatives who must travel to and from the hospital in order to visit the hospitalized patient. When the direct price of care is zero, these transportation costs in comparison with the expected mortality costs discussed above will determine the size of the geographic market.

Conceptually, the relevant geographic market is comprised of all sellers of a particular product line among which the cross-price elasticity of demand for buyers is relatively high. A patient or his physician-agent might seek alternative providers of a particular medical procedure within a geographic market in response to price differentials, but would not seek alternative providers outside of the geographic market. The size of the geographic market depends on the importance and cost of the medical procedure, relative to the travel costs associated with seeking care and the expected mortality costs. These concepts are consistent with markets for some medical procedures being a local metropolitan area, while other procedures could have geographic markets which are regional, national, or even global in scope.

The 1984 Merger Guidelines approach the geographic market as follows:

> the Department seeks to identify a geographic area such that a hypothetical firm that was the only present or future producer or seller of the relevant product in that area could profitably impose a small but significant and nontransitory increase in price. That is, assuming that buyers could respond to a price increase within a tentatively identified area only by shifting to firms located outside the area, what would happen? If firms located elsewhere readily could provide the relevant product to the hypothetical firm's buyers in sufficient quantity at a comparable price, an attempt to raise price would not prove profitable, and the tentatively identified geographic area would prove to be too narrow (1984 Merger Guidelines, p. 13).

This approach is similar to the approach used for the product market definition, as discussed previously, and follows the economic concept of cross-price elasticity quite closely. Further, the Justice Department approach to market definition, since it relies on competitors' response to a price increase, requires that both product and geographic market dimensions be considered in measuring the response.

For hospital mergers, the determination of the relevant geographic market requires examining each economically significant medical procedure to determine geographic market boundaries. Routine procedures such as appendectomies would be expected to have smaller geographic markets than more complex or life-threatening procedures (e.g., plastic surgery, open heart surgery, heart transplants), because the magnitude of transportation costs and expected mortality costs relative to medical costs are lower for the former. To the extent that medical costs are borne by third-party payers, however, the geographic markets may be affected by quality-of-care considerations to a greater extent than price considerations.

IV. THE 1982 AND 1984 JUSTICE DEPARTMENT MERGER GUIDELINES

A. Provisions of the Guidelines

The first Justice Department merger guidelines, announced in 1968, reflected an early effort by the antitrust enforcers to reduce the uncertainty experienced by firms contemplating merger regarding the applicability of the antimerger laws. The relevant statute is Section 7 of the Clayton Act, as amended, which provides:

> That no corporation engaged in commerce shall acquire, directly or indirectly, the whole or any part of the stock or other share capital and no corporation subject to the jurisdiction of the Federal Trade Commission shall acquire the whole or any part of the assets of another corporation engaged also in commerce, where in any line of commerce in any section of the country, the effect of such acquisition may be substantially to lessen competition, or to tend to create a monopoly.

A crucial point of controversy in interpreting the Clayton Act is related to the phrase "where the effect . . . may be substantially to lessen competition, or to tend to create a monopoly." For a 20-year period following the Cellar–Kefauver amendments of 1950, the U.S. Supreme Court took a strict view toward mergers, and most horizontal mergers challenged by the FTC or the Justice Department were disallowed. Conglomerate mergers became the dominant form of merger during the late 1960s and 1970s, partly because case precedent suggested that such mergers were much less likely to be challenged by the antitrust authorities. The arrival of the Reagan administration in 1981 marked an abrupt shift in antitrust policy, reflecting an idealogy which looked with favor on large firms and viewed large size as an indication of efficiency and business success.

This philosophical change is reflected in the 1982 and 1984 merger guidelines (U.S. Department of Justice, 1982 and 1984). Since the two sets of guidelines are similar in most respects, the discussion here is limited to the 1984 guidelines. The guidelines provide a relatively rigorous approach to market definition, as discussed earlier, and also provide quantitative market concentration guidelines which are applicable to horizontal mergers. The intent appears to be both to provide a more systematic approach to the analysis of mergers and to recognize the possibility that some mergers may be procompetitive.

The quantitative market concentration guidelines are based on the Herfindahl–Hirschman Index, referred to as the HHI. This index is a summary measure of market concentration and is defined as follows:

$$HHI = \Sigma s_i^2,$$

where s is the market share of the ith firm in the market. This index, bounded by 0 and 10,000 when market shares are measured in percentages, reflects the complete size distribution of firms in the market, but gives much greater weight to firms with high market shares. For example, in a market with only four firms, if the firms each have a 25% market share, the HHI is 2500, while if the firms' respective shares are 50%, 30 %, 10%, and 10%, the HHI is 3600.

The quantitative guidelines, in general terms, are as follows:

1. If the postmerger HHI is less than 1000 in the relevant market, the Justice Department is unlikely to challenge the merger, except in unusual circumstances.
2. If the postmerger HHI lies between 1000 and 1800, the Department will consider the merger more closely. In this range of the HHI, if the merger causes an increase in the HHI of more than 100 points, the Department is more likely to challenge the merger than if the increase is less than 100 points. Other factors, such as ease of market entry, become more important to the evaluation in this range.
3. If the postmerger HHI exceeds 1800, and if the increase in the HHI due to the merger is more than 50 points, the Department is likely to challenge the merger. Even in such instances, however, other relevant factors will be considered.

The guidelines include foreign trade effects in defining relevant markets, which represents a departure from most previous antitrust practice. The nature of hospital markets, however, makes the feature of the guidelines relatively unimportant except perhaps in markets near national borders.

More important for hospital mergers is the consideration which the guidelines give to efficiencies. The guidelines provide that

> [s]ome mergers that the Department might otherwise challenge may be reasonably necessary to achieve significant net efficiencies. If the parties to the merger establish by clear and convincing evidence that a merger will achieve such efficiencies, the Department will consider those efficiencies in deciding whether to challenge the merger. (U.S. Department of Justice, 1984)

Although efficiencies do not constitute a defense in an otherwise anticompetitive merger, they can effect the probability that a merger will be challenged.

B. Applications of the Guidelines and Relevance to Hospital Markets

In an early application of the 1982 Guidelines, the Justice Department challenged an acquisition by LTV–Republic Steel, based on the HHI in certain product markets within the broad line of steel products. In a subsequent decision, the Department approved a modified merger which included some divestiture provisions. Those divestitures came in market segments in which the HHI exceeded 1800.

The Justice Department and the FTC have joint jurisdiction in enforcement of the Clayton Act prohibitions of anticompetitive mergers. In practice, the agencies tend to have somewhat different enforcement approaches. The FTC has had jurisdiction over the two most recent merger actions brough by the federal authorities (*AMI*, decided in 1984, and *Hospital Corp. of America*, decided in 1985.) In both cases, the FTC decision refers to the HHI index in the context of the Justice Department guidelines in arriving at the conclusion that market concentration in the relevant market is quite high. This small sample of cases suggests that the Justice Department's merger guidelines will have a prominent role in merger proceedings, regardless of which agency brings the action.

Mergers are an important means of market entry by for-profit firms in today's health care marketplace. As the structure of health care markets continues its rapid evolution, this strategy is likely to become even more important. In the likely event that antitrust action may becomes a means of defense against takeover used by the target firm, the guidelines may act to provide a strong defense argument in such civil suits.

V. MARKET CONCENTRATION AND MARKET DEFINITION IN THE 1985 HCA CASE

In 1981, Hospital Corporation of America (HCA) acquired Hospital Affiliates International (HAI) in a $650 million stock acquisition (*Hospital Corp. of America*, CCH Trade Regulation Reports, para. 22,301, 1985). HAI had owned or managed five acute care hospitals in the Chattanooga, Tennessee, area prior to the merger. About four months later, HCA acquired Health Care Corporation (HCC), which owned one acute care hospital in Chattanooga. As a result of these acquisitions, HCA increased its market position in the Chattanooga metropolitan statistical area from ownership of one acute care hospital to ownership or management of 7 of the 14 hospitals in the area.

The FTC challenged the merger, and in an administrative law judge's opinion, which was largely upheld by the FTC upon appeal, the defendant was found in violation of the Clayton Act and was required to divest some of its hospital units in the Chattanooga area. Of particular interest in this case are the approach used in defining the relevant product and geographic markets and the FTC's general approach of finding the Clayton Act applicable to hospital markets, despite their somewhat unusual institutional characteristics.

The administrative law judge in the HCA case defined the relevant product market to be "the cluster of services offered by acute care hospitals, including outpatient as well as inpatient care. . . . " The judge excluded the outpatient services provided by nonhospital institutions, pointing to the unique combination of services which the acute care patient needs (*Hospital Corp. of America*, Section III). The FTC decision considers whether or not nonhospital providers should be included in the relevant product market, but makes no clear reference to the possibility that the relevant product market is at the procedure or diagnosis level rather than including the broad cluster of hospital services.

In considering the relevant geographic market, the HCA proceedings included consideration of patient flow data which identified the origin of patients. Although there was some disagreement over whether the relevant geographic market area was the urban area of Chattanooga or the broader metropolitan area, the FTC decision chose the narrower urban area. The decision pointed out the need to consider the likelihood that patients and physicians would travel to outlying hospitals, given the high times costs of the associated travel.

With respect to market concentration, the HHI index in the Chattanooga urban area was in the 1900–2200 range before the mergers and in the 2400–2600 range after both mergers had been carried out. These concentration levels were a major piece of evidence in this case, especially when considered in conjunction with relatively high entry barriers and the traditional tendency for hospitals to avoid direct price competition.

The Commission concluded that the effect of the qcquisitions "may be substantially to lessen competition in the Chattanooga urban area general acute care hospital market." The respondent presented two defenses: first, the uniqueness of the health care market and implied immunity; and second, efficiencies resulting from the merger. Both of these lines of defense were rejected by the FTC.

The 1985 HCA decision is a rather strong affirmation by the federal antitrust enforcers that hospital mergers will be subjected to the same antitrust scrutiny as mergers in other more conventional product markets. The relevant geographic market for hospital mergers is generally the local urban area, with patient flow data and travel cost considerations important in deciding the scope of the geographic market.

VI. METHODS OF ANALYSIS AND DATA

Only a few studies have directly addressed the notion of competition between hospitals. Luft and Maerki (1984/85) developed measures of hospital clusters using predetermined measures of distances of 5 and 15 miles between (presumed) hospital locations. They concluded, based on these distance measures, that a substantial number of hospitals do not have potential competitors nearby. However, they did not test the validity of their assumptions with actual patient flow data, and so the actual distribution of the degree of the degree of competition in the various markets is unknown.

Joskow (1980) developed Herfindahl (H) Indexes on the size distribution of hospital beds within SMSAs. For hospitals in rural areas he assumed a value of H of 1 (equivalent to value of 10,000 for the HHI). Joskow also used two other variables to measure competition—a measure of physician–

hospital concentration and one of the impact of HMOs in the market. Farley (1985) developed Herfindahl Indexes using hospital gross capital stock with counties as the relevant market area. Farley assumed that a value for H of ⅕ or less signified a competitive market, while a value of 1 was monopolistic. An intermediate group fell in between. As with Luft and Maerki, neither Joskow nor Farley determined the validity of their assumed measures.

Our analysis of hospital market competition measures is based on countywide counts of hospital inpatients for specific diagnoses. We should stress that our measure of patient flows is all the residents of each county for the specific diagnosis who were discharged from any hospital in South Carolina.

The data base comes from discharge abstracts for all inpatient cases for each South Carolina hospital in 1980. The data are collected annually by the South Carolina Cooperative Health Statistics project of the state's Budget and Control Board. Product lines were based on diagnostic and procedure groupings for selected major surgical procedures and all non-surgical cases (by ICDA-9 major groups).

All discharges of residents of each market area in diagnosis A who were discharged from Hospital i (called D_i) were tabulated. Also tabulated were all discharges of diagnosis A for all residents (i.e., from all hospitals) who were discharged (called D). The market area Herfindahl index was calculated for each diagnosis as

$$H = \Sigma \left(\frac{D_i}{D}\right)^2,$$

where the summation is over all South Carolina hospitals serving patients who were residents of that market area. Omitted from this measure were patients who went out of state; this appears to be a problem for only a few, highly specialized procedures and for two counties bordering Charlotte, North Carolina, and Augusta, Georgia.

VII. RESULTS

This section presents the results of calculating H indexes using the methods described in the previous section.

Further, we will concentrate on surgical procedures only, because they appear to represent more clearly defined product lines.

For purposes of discussing antitrust issues, we focus our attention on two representative geographic markets in South Carolina: the Columbia SMSA, consisting of two counties with four general hospitals; and the Orangeburg County market, a non-SMSA with a single general hospital. These two markets represent the extremes in expected market concentration as typified in the cited literature.

Table 1.   Area Herfindahl Values by Diagnosis

Diagnosis	Columbia Metro	Orangeburg County
All diagnoses	2600	2600
Obstetrics	3300	6200
Surgical procedures (total)	2400	4600
Nervous system	4600	1700
Ophthalmology	4400	2400
Otorhinolaryngology	2600	4400
Tonsillectomy/adenoidectomy	2400	6100
Thyroid/thymus	2700	5500
Vascular/cardiac	3000	2400
Thoracic	2800	3800
Abdominal	2700	5000
Hernia repair	2800	6100
Appendectomy	2800	7000
Cholecystectomy	3200	6100
Procto-surgery	2800	6200
Urological	2700	5500
Breast	3000	4400
Gynecological	3600	3700
Orthopedic	3600	5300
Plastic surgery	2300	1700
Oral/maxillofacial	2600	2100
Dental	4200	1300
Other	2900	4400

The results are summarized in Table 1. Somewhat contrary to conventional wisdom, both the metropolitan area market and the rural county market exhibit the same *overall* degree of competition: the value of H in both cases is 2600. These values are roughly the same order of magnitude as those in the Chattanooga market as cited in the FTC's *Hospital Corp. of America* decision (1985). In both cases the overall value of H is greater than the 1800 level which the Justice Department guidelines suggest to be the critical level.

At the individual procedure level, which we believe in many cases to be the relevant product market, the degree of concentration varies widely. For example, in the metropolitan area market, the concentration measures for surgical procedures range from 2300 (plastic surgery) to 4600 (nervous system operations). There is no clear relationship between procedure complexity and the value of H. For the rural county, the range of H is much greater: from 1700 (nervous system) to 7000 (appendectomy). Curiously, the more complicated procedures in this market tend to have the *lower* concentration levels.

Table 1 presents us with a paradox. On the one hand, aggregate levels of concentration in the metropolitan and rural markets are equal. On the other hand, there are considerable differences in concentration measures for individual procedures. Furthermore, some procedures in the rural county, where competition would be expected to be minimal, are associated with lower H measures than in the metropolitan area.

An explanation for this is that the hospital product market cannot be considered in isolation from the geographic market. For some procedures the geographic market is wider than for others: as the procedure becomes more complex, the probability that a given hospital will offer that procedure decreases. In rural areas, with one or two smaller hospitals, patients needing these procedures frequently travel to larger hospitals outside what would appear to be the geographic market. This would account for lower values of H for the more complex procedures in the rural county, since once patients leave the rural county, the range of alternatives is broader than a single metropolitan area.

If those leaving the county for treatment go to different hospitals for different procedures, then the *aggregate* measured value of H may give the appearance of a high degree of competition. In fact, regarding competition in hospital care as an aggregate cluster of services masks the varied patterns of patient travel in what are, in effect, different procedure markets.

Another way of looking at this problem is to relate it to the definition of the relevant geographic market. A proposed test for a geographic market is to look at the flow of customers into and out of the proposed market area (Elzinga and Hogarty, 1973). An appropriately defined geographic market would have small percentages of customers flowing in each direction. The data shown in Table 2 provide measures of patient flows into and out of the Columbia SMSA market and the Orangeburg county market, for all inpatient cases and for selected surgical procedures. Overall, the Columbia data show that defining the SMSA as the relevant geographic market may provide too narrow a definition. But this conclusion will in fact vary considerably by procedure. For example, 46% of all cardiac surgery cases in Columbia SMSA hospitals come from outside the SMSA area; the figure for appendectomies is only 10.8%.

Referring to the Orangeburg market, overall the county is not a good measure of the geographic market. And, in fact, for more complicated procedures (ophthalmologic surgery, cardiac surgery) the majority of cases leave the county. However, for less complicated procedures (appendectomy) the county definition may be acceptable.

The general impression one receives from the data shown in Tables 1 and 2 is that there are important differences in the degree of competition across surgical procedures which conventional approaches would place in the same relevant geographic and product market. In the Columbia market,

Table 2.   Patient Flows to and from Columbia SMSA and Orangeburg
County Hospitals

Diagnosis Group	Percent of Columbia SMSA Resident Patients Who Go Out of SMSA	Percent of Orangeburg County Resident Patients Who Go Out of County	Percnet of Columbia SMSA Hospital Pattents Who Are Non-SMSA Residents	Percent of Orangeburg Hospital Patients Who Are Out-of-County Residents
Total	2.8%	26.6%	20.4%	23.5%
Obstetrics	1.1	20.8	14.1	21.4
Surgical procedures	2.9	31.0	22.2	27.4
Nervous system	4.2	81.9	33.6	23
Ophthalmology	4.0	59.5	27.1	34.8
Otorhinolaryngology	7.7	26.3	23.8	20.3
Tonsillectomy/adenoidectomy	4.3	21.2	14.9	20.4
Thyroid/thymus	2.7	26.8	18.2	25
Vascular/cardiac	5.1	61.7	46	20.4
Thoracic	2.6	38.1	28.6	28.8
Abdominal	2.0	28.1	20.1	22
Hernia repair	1.3	18.8	13.5	27.3
Appendectomy	3.1	12.9	10.8	19.2
Cholecystectomy	0.6	21.9	13.1	23.6
Procto-surgery	1.8	17.8	13.5	27.8
Urological	2.5	23.9	17.0	36.5
Breast	1.7	34.4	16.4	19.1
Gynecological	1.4	16.8	14	27.5
Orthopedic	3.5	27.6	20.6	32.7
Plastic surgery	5.8	68.8	23.5	39.1
Oral/maxillofacial	9.0	60.7	20.9	21.4
Dental	0.3	78.5	21.3	0
Other	2.1	31.4	17	20.7

actual market concentration measured at the procedure level tends to be higher than overall market concentration. In the Orangeburg market, actual market concentration at the procedure level is higher than overall concentration, but lower than the total monopoly level that would be suggested by conventional analysis. Generally, these empirical results support the argument that market concentration in hospital markets should be measured at the diagnosis or procedure level.

The geography of South Carolina is such that travel costs between rural and urban areas are not great. A number of other states have similar population dispersions, and we believe that our results can be generalized to these states. In all probability, there are some rural areas in the West where patient travel costs are much higher, and therefore for these states referral patterns may be different.

VIII. CONCLUSIONS

The mere fact that antitrust policy toward hospital mergers is a topic of current interest is an indication of the major changes that have occurred in the markets for health care services. Not long ago, the topic would have been irrelevant, both because most hospitals were publicly owned, and because the health care sector was largely considered exempt from the antitrust laws. The current interest in the topic reflects the increased participation of the private sector in the hospital industry as well as the increasing importance of competition in the operating environments of hospitals.

As hospitals seek to enter new markets and consolidate existing markets, merger will continue to be an attractive means of market entry. The representative levels of the HHI observed in the South Carolina markets discussed in this paper, considered against the merger guidelines suggested by the U.S. Justice Department, suggest that hospital mergers in many markets are likely to be difficult to carry out without attracting the attention of the antitrust enforcers.

The observed differences across surgical procedures in the level of market concentration and in the scope of the geographic market are consistent with the argument that the relevant product market for hospitals is at the individual procedure, rather than at the broad cluster of services level. This approach to the analysis of hospital competition will become even more important in the future as nonhospital providers become more viable.

REFERENCES

Alpert, Geraldine and McCarthy, Thomas R. (1984), "Beyond Goldfarb: Applying Traditional Antitrust Analysis to Changing Health Markets." *The Antitrust Bulletin* 39(2):165–204.

Blair, Roger D. and Kaserman, David L. (1985), *Antitrust Economics*. Homewood, IL: Irwin.

Bronsteen, Peter (1984), "A Review of the Revised Merger Guidelines." *The Antitrust Bulletin* 39(4):613–652.

Brozen, Yale (1982), *Mergers in Perspective*. Washington, DC: American Enterprise Institute.

Christianson, Jon B. (1984), "Provider Participation in Competitive Bidding for Indigent Patients." *Inquiry* 21:161–177.

Farley, Dean E. (1985), *Competition Among Hospitals*. Hospital Studies Program, Hospital Cost and Utilization Project, Research Note 7. Rockville, MD: National Center for Health Services Research and Health Care Technology Assessment, U.S. Department of Health and Human Services, Publication (PHS) 85-3353.

Fox, Eleanor M. and Halverson, James T., eds. (1984), *Antitrust Policy in Transition: The Convergence of Law and Economics*. New York: American Bar Association.

Frech, H. E. and Paul B. Ginsburg (1975), "Imposed Health Insurance in Monopolistic Markets." *Economic Inquiry* 13(1): 55-70.

Goldfarb, Marsha, Mark Hornbrook, and John Rafferty (1980), "Behavior of the Multi-product Firm." *Medical Care* 18(2):185–201.

Joskow, Paul L. (1980), "The Effects of Competition and Regulation on Hospital Bed Supply and Reservation Quality of the Hospital." *Bell Journal of Economics* 11(2):421–447.

Lave, Judith R., and Lester B. Lave (1984). "Hospital Cost Functions." *Annual Review of Public Health* 5:193–213.

Luft, Harold S., J. P. Bunker, and A. C. Enthoven (1979), "Should Operations be Region-alized?" *New England Journal of Medicine* 301:1364–1369.

Luft, Harold S. and Susan C. Maerki (1984/85), "Competitive Potential of Hospitals and Their Neighbors." *Contemporary Policy Issues* 3(1):89–102.

Mason, Scott A. (1979), "The Multihospital Movement Defined." *Public Health Reports* 94(5):446–453.

Posner, Richard A. (1976), *Antitrust Law: An Economic Perspective*. Chicago: University of Chicago Press.

Salkever, David and Thomas W. Bice (1976), "The Impact of Certificate of Need Controls on Hospital Investments." *Milbank Memorial Fund Quarterly* pp.185–214.

Scherer, F. Michael (1980), *Industrial Market Structure and Economic Performance*, 2nd ed. Chicago: Rand McNally.

Schramm, Carl J. and Steven C. Penn, "Hospital Mergers, Market Concentration and the Herfindahl–Hirschman Index." *Emory Law Journal* 33(4):869–888.

U.S. Department of Justice (1984), Merger Guidelines. Reprinted in Commerce Clearing House, *Trade Regulation Reports*, No. 655.

U.S. Federal Trade Commission (1982), "Statement of Federal Trade Commission Con-cerning Horizontal Mergers." Reprinted in *Trade Regulation Reports*, 546:71–87.

U.S. Federal Trade Commission (1984), Final Order to Cease and Desist, American Medical International et al. *Trade Regulation Reports*, para. 22,170.

U.S. Federal Trade Commission (1985), Final Order to Cease and Desist, Hospital Corp. of America. *Trade Regulation Reports*, para. 22,301.

White, William D. (1979), "Regulating Competition in a Nonprofit Industry." *Inquiry* 16:50–61.

COMMENTS ON ANTITRUST ISSUES

H. E. Frech III

Both papers presented in Part III of this volume cover important issues for antitrust in the hospital industry. The paper by Roger Blair and James Fesmire presents a fine review of the antitrust law and economics of mergers and then makes two related policy arguments. First, drawing heavily on Clark's excellent but oddly neglected *Harvard Law Review* paper, they claim that the nonprofit legal form is no longer appropriate for hospitals. Flowing from that, they argue that mergers of nonprofit hospitals should not be given preferential treatment under the antitrust laws. The contribution by Philip Jacobs and Ronald Wilder is less philosophical. Rather, it gives a nuts-and-bolts treatment of how one should go about defining markets and measuring market shares for hospital antitrust.

While both papers are worthwhile and stimilating, I find myself sympathetic to the economic and policy analysis of Blair and Fesmire, but not so sympathetic to the details of the approach to market definition taken by Jacobs and Wilder. Let me discuss Blair and Fesmire first.

Missing in the list of motives for hospital merger is the possibility of reducing nonprice competition. Early results from a research project con-

Advances in Health Economics and Health Services Research, Vol. 7, pgs. 263–267.
Copyright © 1987 by JAI Press Inc.
All rights of reproduction in any form reserved.
ISBN: 0-89232-573-9

ducted by Michael Woolley and me indicate that where there are fewer competing hospitals, both price competition and nonprice competition are affected. Specifically, where there are fewer hospitals, costs decline substantially as nonprice competition is less vigorous. However, with fewer hospitals, price competition is so attenuated that prices decline less. Weaker price competition prevents the lower costs from being passed on to consumers. Thus, the price of quality-adjusted hospital days would rise as the number of hospitals in a market declined. I was encouraged to find that these early results have been corroborated by a study of a different data set by Monica Noether at the Federal Trade Commission.

If so, hospitals merging to increase market power are likely to expect that their merger will have little effect on hospital prices, but will allow them to raise margins and profits by decreasing quality and amenities.

Blair's and Fesmire's discussion of merger that results in a more concentrated oligopoly suggests that the only consumer welfare problem is that collusion is easier to establish and maintain in more concentrated markets. However, this is only part of the problem. Many, perhaps most, oligopoly models predict higher prices as concentration rises. Examples include the standard models of Cournot and Stackelberg. Thus, even with independent behavior, one would expect mergers that raise concentration to lead to higher prices, at least if the post-merger concentration is high enough.

The paper attributes the easing of antitrust enforcement generally that has occurred in recent years at the Justice Department and the Federal Trade Commission to a new political attitude that is more favorable to the business sector. I disagree. A genuine scientific revolution has occurred that affects our economic and legal understanding of monopoly and oligopoly behavior, which has led to a more thoughtful and rational approach to antitrust. It is difficult to trace all of the intellectual roots of the revolution, but it is clear that the early work of Aaron Director and Edward Levi at the University of Chicago was one source. Whatever the many sources of the original ideas, the revolution has spread far and wide and now includes such people as Michael Spence at Harvard, Oliver Williamson at Yale, Bobby Willig at Princeton, Rick Warren-Boulton at the Justice Department and even Roger Blair at Florida. The revolution has also profoundly influenced, if not converted, such defenders of the old guard as my friend and colleague Bill Comanor.

Blair and Fesmire are silent on why nonprofit hospitals came to dominate the industry if they are inherently less efficient. I believe that the answer is historical, as argued by William White and Peter Temin (the latter in an unpublished essay). Most hospitals were founded in the nineteenth century as charitable institutions for the poor only. Middle-class consumers were treated at home. These early hospitals were almost totally dependent on private or local government donations for support. The nonprofit form of property right was a useful protection for the donors, especially small donors. By attenuating the claim of those in control to the profits or residual, the nonprofit legal form prevented donations from going directly into the stockholders' pockets. In the twentieth century, this all changed. Hospitals became businesses. By now, they receive almost no donations, but rather supply servies for which middle-class consumers are more than willing to pay. For most modern hospitals, the nonprofit form is anachronistic.

I agree with the authors that the performance of nonprofit hospitals is inferior to that of profit-seeking ones. However, Frank Sloan and others have shown that the differences are very small, both for efficiency and willingness to treat nonpaying consumers. I think that there are two reasons for this. First, competition for consumers among nonprofit hospitals is and has been important. Competition in the output market has prevented the worst excesses of nonprofit inefficiency. Second, the external incentives of cost reimbursement and very complete insurance (with small or no copayment) have given hospitals with both kinds of property rights little reason to pursue efficiency. Several recent developments in the public and private insurance market promise to change this situation.

The Medicare disease diagnosis-related group (DRG) hospital reimbursement system has already improved incentives somewhat and probably will continue to do so. More important are developments in the private insurance market. Both growing preferred provider organizations (PPOs) and rising consumer copayments will dramatically improve incentives. Under these more appropriate incentives, both profit-seeking and nonprofit hospitals will perform better, with an increasing advantage to the profit-seeking hospitals. Except for the occasional research-oriented institution, nonprofit hospitals will pattern themselves closely after the profit-seeking hospitals in order to survive.

Blair and Fesmire devote little attention to market definition issues. But, their views appear to be very similar to those of Jacobs and Wilder, so I will not discuss them separately here.

Regarding Jacobs and Wilder's paper, I want to go back to the fundamental definition of a market for antitrust purposes. The issue is: Which sellers can constrain the higher prices or lower quality of a colluding group of other sellers? For example, if Hospitals A and B cannot profitably collude to significantly raise price and/or reduce quality for a significant time period, then it must be the case that the competition of other hospitals constrains their behavior. If so, these other hospitals should be included in the market. The market definition problem is to determine which sellers to include in the analysis.

The U.S. Justice Department's merger guidelines have made an excellent contribution in two ways. First, they focused the theory on the right central idea—the ability of other sellers to constrain monopolistic behavior. Second, they made more concrete the idea of a "significant" price increase and time period. The guidelines suggest that a 5% price rise for one year is significant. The market is the smallest number of sellers who could collude to raise price by 5% for one year. It some mergers, the relevant market could be as small as the two hospitals who are merging.

The idea of substitution is subsidiary. One investigates substitution only to determine the constraining effect of some sellers on a particular group of sellers. Jacobs and Wilder's discussion of substitution in demand by consumers is fine. However, they neglected the issue of substitution in supply by sellers. And this led them astray. Even if there were no possible substitution in demand between the products of two different sellers, easy substitution in supply would require that the sellers of the disparate goods be included in the same relevant market. The classic example is the machine tool industry. Most of the products are not very substitutable in use (e.g., milling machines, lathes, automatic screw machines). However, the manufacturers can easily shift from one line of goods to another, so they are all included in the machine tool industry.

Applying this principle to produce market definition for hospitals, we see that hospitals can easily shift resources from one procedure or diagnosis to another, even though the procedures and services (e.g., eye surgery and appendectomies) are not at all substitutable in consumption. Further, many hospital services are strong complements to each other. Hotel services, meals, blood tests, X-rays and surgery are all necessary to produce an inpatient surgical service. Thus, the relevant product market for hospitals should be viewed as the cluster of services provided in hospitals. The hundred or thousands of individual procedures or services should not be viewed as individual markets.

There may be some rare services where certificate-of-need regulation or scale economies make it difficult for some hospitals to begin to sell the service. Still, it is usually best to ignore these. First, mergers or collusion are unlikely to affect the number of sellers of such rare services. Second, where scale economies are the problem, all hospitals present potential competition to be the one hospital that actually provides the service. Of course, if two hospitals providing these unusual services do merge, this merger is worse for competition than most.

One implication of my view is that outpatient care centers should be excluded from the relevant hospital market. While there has been substantial movement of care from inpatient to outpatient settings, especially for surgery, we must not infer that they are close substitutes in the economic sense. That is, consumers may not be willing to change from inpatient to outpatient care in response to a small price rise for inpatient care. The actual reasons for the movement of care outside the hospital appear to be the availability of the care on an outpatient basis for those who preferred it that way all along and extreme forms of insurer pressure (e.g., no benefits for minor surgery done on an inpatient basis) for others. Outpatient services do not much constrain inpatient prices.

Turning to geographic markets, one needs to be careful in interpreting data on travel for hospital care. In particular, the willingness of some consumers to travel long distances for nonprice reasons does not mean that distant hospitals should be included in the relevant geographic market. Santa Barbara consumers are unlikely to be much influenced on whether or not to go to Stanford or UCLA because of a small change in Santa Barbara hospital prices. Small price changes at the famous research hospitals are equally unlikely to cause many consumers to change their choices about outmigration for sophisticated hospital care.

Patient origin data should also be handled with care. One would like to find a geographic boundary enclosing a particular group of sellers such that those sellers comprise the market. Patient origin data that showed little outmigration and little inmigration for hospital care would be one piece of evidence that one has found a relevant economic market. But this is only one piece of evidence. And a group of sellers with substantial in and outmigration may still be a market if the migration appears to be occurring in response to nonprice variables, as discussed above. Of course, it is very helpful if there are natural boundaries, such as farmland, rivers, or mountains, separating groups of sellers. In large homogeneous metropolitan areas, it may be very difficult to define geographic boundaries.

PART IV:

SUMMARY AND REFLECTIONS

MERGERS IN HEALTH CARE
IMPLICATIONS FOR THE FUTURE

Allen Dobson

I. INTRODUCTION

The conference at which the papers in this volume were delivered was an extraordinary one. I choose these words deliberately because much of the conventional wisdom related to the eventual impact of changing market structures in the health care marketplace was challenged there. Because change is so predominant in health care today, perhaps this should come as little surprise. It is difficult to predict future market structures, let alone surmise the implications these market structures will have for the performance of future health care delivery systems. The clear value of this conference, though, was not only its questioning of this current knowledge base and outlook, but also its provision of a new set of facts. Properly arranged, this set of facts might constitute a framework to help us more precisely interpret the long-run implications of change as it occurs. As our science is not particularly adept at either predicting turning points in time series or understanding their immediate consequences, the framework developed at this conference may be particularly useful.

Advances in Health Economics and Health Services Research, Vol. 7, pgs. 271–277.
Copyright © 1987 by JAI Press Inc.
All rights of reproduction in any form reserved.
ISBN: 0-89232-573-9

What I would like to do herein is to first provide a broad context for interpreting the conference's papers. By observing the historical preconditions for today's changes, perhaps we can better understand findings as they become available. Given this perspective, I will then summarize results across the various papers. Finally, I will comment on the degree to which health care services research is likely to impact on public policy during a time when one set of health care policies is barely understood before a new set is implemented.

II. A BRIEF HISTORICAL PERSPECTIVE

There are several historical trends of growth and expansion that are pertinent to today's discussion: These include the growth and development of—

- Reimbursement, coverage, eligibility, and health care insurance administrative policies since the 1930s
- The supply of hospitals (and other institutional providers) and the supply of physicians—as influenced by insurance coverage, tax policy, and government intervention such as Hill–Burton and manpower legislation
- Public programs, particularly Medicare and Medicaid, which have augmented the private insurance industry in the removal of price as a consideration in the medical marketplace; and
- Health care services research, in terms of research capability and influence on public policy

The interaction of these key developments has resulted in the preconditions for today's changing environment and our understanding of health care delivery evolution. Research in the 1920s and 1930s lead to the perception that if supply was enhanced, not only would access increase but prices, if not expenditures, would fall. The current "oversupply" of physicians may be the first true embodiment of these early speculations. Before the recent surge in physicians, however, the growth of the private insurance and hospital industries—augmented by government and union–employers' policies—set the building blocks of our current health care delivery system in place during the 1950s and 1960s.

By 1965, with the enactment of Medicare and Medicaid, access issues for most of the population were well on their way to being solved. Yet, as early as 1967, expenditures were becoming a primary legislative concern, and by the early 1970s regulatory cost containment mechanisms were legislated and implemented. (It is interesting to note that even as these reforms were being implemented, Medicare was expanded to include the disabled and end-stage renal disease populations.) Despite the initiation of these regulatory activities, response in the marketplace went unabated. Expenditures continued to rise at unprecedented rates (aside from a brief respite engendered by wage and price controls). The inflationary incentives inherent in restrospective cost-based reimbursement proved far too strong for professional standards review organizations (PSROs), certificates of need (CONs), planning authorities, and various reimbursement limit systems.

The upshot of a half-century of public and private policy development was an "oversupply" of hospitals and doctors and a provider industry very sophisticated at extracting revenues from existing reimbursement systems. From the early 1970s to the early 1980s, expenditures rose by nearly 20% annually and, all things considered, policy changed at a leisurely pace given the problems at hand.

By 1983, however, the rules of the game were to change dramatically. Health care services research clearly uncovered the failures of policies of the 1970s. Yet, three promising solutions to these failures were also emerging. The first was that demonstrations with prospective payment at the State and local level, culminating with the New Jersey diagnosis-related groups (DRGs) experiment, suggested that prospective pricing represented a powerful system of incentives that could result in expenditures control. The current Medicare prospective payment system (PPS) would be subsequently derived from this body of research and demonstrations. The second was the move by the insurance industry to various systems of managed care and an almost universal increase in cost-sharing provisions. At the same time, employers responded with a series of cost-containment initiatives. The third was the interest and willingness of a more diversified set of players to absorb the underwriting function. Health maintenance organizations (HMOs) became risk takers, as did some insurance companies and employers.

The consequence of these changes in incentives has proved nothing less than dramatic. Public and private initiatives have resulted in fewer hospital admissions and generally more efficient use of health care services. The health care market has shifted rapidly from a seller's market to a buyer's market in both the public and private sectors. Purchasers are no longer willing to let providers dictate the levels of supply and prices for health care.

In the mid-1980s, the cycle of change has become both more rapid—as noted by the incredible change in provider and payor behavior since 1983— and more complex, as marked by the fact that institutions are changing very rapidly as they adapt to new marketplace incentives.

Is it any wonder that various glimpses of this virtual revolution are seemingly contradictory and that our measurement and analytic techniques are not entirely up to the task? Health care services research was not designed to measure revolutions. It is difficult enough to understand evolution. As I will note below, the main threads of health care services research—access, quality, and cost—will remain central to our work. Yet these papers strongly suggest that it is time we expand our collective horizons and attempt to determine the exact nature and the resulting implications of a rapidly changing health care services market structure. My suspicion after reading these papers is that many of our old notions of market structure results will need to be refined and revised as new facts emerge.

III.   AN OVERVIEW OF CONFERENCE RESULTS

A.   Characteristics of Mergers

The authors have been able to describe the characteristics of mergers reasonably well. Mergers appear to be occurring relatively rapidly, but not as fast as common wisdom would have us believe. The impression we are left with is that thus far relatively small numbers of hospitals are involved, but that more are surely to merge in the future. More quantification would be useful in this regard.

Hospitals seem to acquire and merge with similar types of hospitals in terms of ownership. As a result, the for-profit hospitals do not seem to be taking over the health care marketplace, as many would have us believe.

Yet mergers do have at least two broad marketplace implications:

- If there is to be a health industrial complex it will take a different form than previously predicted as nonprofit organizations start to emulate for-profit ones.
- Often, there are fewer beds after merger than there were before, and mergers seem to take place in the same market area. There is little evidence presented in these papers that national chains are the norm in the merger process. Indeed, if we can believe our case study of one, the merger model is likely to be one of transition from individual competitors to horizontal mergers to vertical integration, with some amount of underwriting function being assumed by hospitals and other health care providers along the way.

B.   Merger Dynamics

The rationale for mergers we are presented with is less compelling than the discussion of merger characteristics. The notion that mergers improve capital formation is not firmly upheld. Presumably, mergers take place in order to improve economic performance—economies of scale in production, specialization, purchasing power, and the like. Yet the economic performance of the evolving systems does not seem to be noticeably superior to that of single hospitals. Because mergers are based on a priori expectations, it's very difficult to measure the underlying causes of mergers.

In addition to the above characteristics, certain marketplace phenomena seem to be associated with mergers. These include:

- A high proportion of Medicaid revenues
- A high proportion of private insurance
- A favorable attitude by the states toward mergers and investor-owned hospitals
- The fact that investors seem to be very cognizant of the capital rules set forth by payors and to seek out favorable treatment

Certain other variables, however, do not seem to be associated with mergers. These include:

- Competitive environments, as measured by the presence of HMOs
- Bad risks, which apparently are not sought out by good performers, as common wisdom suggest
- Rate setting, which appears to work against mergers (though it will be interesting to see if PPS has this negative effect on mergers)
- Government hospitals, which are more likely to be managed than purchased (in general, though, management contracts are not well explained in these papers)
- Physicians, who apparently have not had a dominant influence on mergers (perhaps, the physician surplus has weakened their relative bargaining position, or perhaps mergers are in the physicians' best interest in terms of coverage and lifestyle)

Presumably, mergers are a response to shifts in market conditions as payors change their behavior. Mergers are seen as a way to insure market penetration (increase market power along product lines) and long-term survival. Could this be the one instance in corporate America where a long-range view of profits and survival is taken, or is this merely a reflection of a broader merger mania ("paper profits")?

We were also not given a very precise picture in these papers of who the purchasers actually are. It is not clear to me how the large chains relate to the small chains in terms of patient load, location, and merger strategy. Our case study of HCA suggests that it is not clear to the chains either, as goals and mission change as rapidly as the latest stock market quotation.

The fact that we could not describe the dynamics of merger is not at all surprising, as economic and social theory is seldom very accurate in predicting "turning points" or change. We rely on historical precedent. As implied above, there is not much of that to work from here.

C. Summary

We can describe mergers in a descriptive fashion, but we do not know very much about merger strategy and rationale. Most importantly, we have not yet determined their impact on competition in the marketplace.

The implications of the consolidating aspects of mergers have obviously not been well thought out. The airline industry is often cited as an example of how deregulation might work in the health care industry. But note the differences. In the airline industry, there are typically more competitors on a given route, not fewer. I suspect the airline industry is a particularly inept analogy to what is happening in health care. While there is much competitive effort being undertaken as consolidation proceeds, consolidation is not always associated with enhanced competition. Enhanced market power through merger and broader control of health care alternatives through vertical integration need to be carefully observed as to eventual competitive effect.

IV. HEALTH CARE SERVICES RESEARCH AND PUBLIC POLICY DURING TRANSITION

From a public policy perspective, health care services research is entering a very difficult time period. It is unlikely that current findings will dramatically alter near-term public policy on mergers and capitation. Yet they do provide a baseline which will help us as we take up the next several tasks of health care services research as they relate to financing.

A. Short-Term Research

As we conduct PPS analyses in view of midcourse corrections, we will need to know more about—

- How to interpret initial high-profit levels, as PPS completes its transition phases
- Access to care
- Changing expenditure level
- Quality of care (the "sicker and quicker" issue)
- The efficiency of health care delivery
- Linkages between payment and severity/intensity

- What happens as fewer resources are put into the health care sector by both private and public funding sources
- How "nonmarket" functions such as uncompensated care, teaching functions, research and the like will be dealt with politically as purchasers become more stringent in their reimbursement practices

The challenge is to be able to detect problems in a timely fashion before they become unmanageable. The papers in this volume can establish the groundwork for future analysis along these lines.

B. Longer-Term Research

As I have said, however, I doubt that current health care services research will help formulate policy for the initial wave of mergers and capitation. It is occurring too fast for us to even record events, let alone influence them. The course for the near term seems pretty well set.

On the other hand, as concentration and capitation evolve, much will need to be done concerning

- Pricing and market determination
- What happens when the incentives are for less care, not more (as was previously the case)
- Uncompensated care

All of this represents a real challenge to health care services research. I hope we can build the bridge between PPS and the competitive/merged/capitated delivery systems of tomorrow. If given the proper support and interest by the citizens of this nation, I think we can.

Research Annuals and Monographs in Series in
BUSINESS, ECONOMICS AND MANAGEMENT

Advances in the Economics of Energy and Resources
Edited by John R. Moroney, *Department of Economics, Texas A & M University*

Applications of Management Science
Edited by Randall L. Schultz, *School of Management, The University of Texas at Dallas*

Perspectives on Local Public Finance and Public Policy
Edited by John M. Quigley, *Graduate School of Public Policy, University of California, Berkeley*

Public Policy and Government Organizations
Edited by John P. Crecine, *College of Humanities and Social Sciences, Carnegie-Mellon University*

Research in Consumer Behavior
Edited by Jagdish N. Sheth, *School of Business, University of Southern California*

Research in Corporate Social Performance and Policy
Edited by Lee E. Preston, *Center for Business and Public Policy, University of Maryland*

Research in Domestic and International Agribusiness Management
Edited by Ray A. Goldenberg, *Graduate School of Business Administration, Harvard University*

Research in Economic History
Edited by Paul Uselding, *Department of Economics, University of Illinois*

Research in Experimental Economics
Edited by Vernon L. Smith, *Department of Economics, University of Arizona*

Research in Finance
Edited by Haim Levy, *School of Business, The Hebrew University and The Wharton School, University of Pennsylvania*

Research in Governmental and Non-Profit Accounting
Edited by James L. Chan, *Department of Accounting, University of Illinois*

Research in Human Captial and Development
Edited by Ismail Sirageldin, *Departments of Population Dynamics and Policital Economy, The Johns Hopkins University*

Research in International Business and Finance
Edited by H. Peter Grey, *Department of Economics, Rutgers University*

Research in International Business and International Relations
Edited by Anant R. Negandhi, *Department of Business Administration, University of Illinois*

Research in Labor Economics
Edited by Ronald G. Ehrenberg, *School of Industrial and Labor Relations, Cornell University*

Research in Law and Economics
Edited by Richard O. Zerbe, Jr., *School of Public Affairs, University of Washington*

Research in Marketing
Edited by Jagdish N. Sheth, *School of Business, University of Southern California*

Research in Organizational Behavior
Edited by Barry M. Staw, *School of Business Administration, University of California, Berkeley* and L.L. Cummings, *J.L. Kellogg Graduate School of Management, Northwestern University*

Research in Personnel and Human Resources Management
Edited by Kendrith M. Rowland, *Department of Business Administration, University of Illinois* and Gerald R. Ferris, *Department of Management, Texas A & M University*

Research in Philosophy and Technology
Edited by Paul T. Durbin, *Philosophy Department and Center for Science and Culture, University at Delaware.* Review and Bibliography Editor: Carl Mitcham, *New York Polytechnic Institute*

Research in Political Economy
Edited by Paul Zarembka, *Department of Economics, State University of New York at Buffalo*

Research in Population Economics
Edited by T. Paul Schultz, *Department of Economics, Yale University* and Kenneth I. Wolpin, *Department of Economics, Ohio State University*

Research in Public Sector Economics
Edited by P.M. Jackson, *Department of Economics, Leicester University*

Research in Real Estate
Edited by C.F. Sirmans, *Department of Finance, Louisiana State University*

Research in the History of Economic Thought and Methodology
Edited by Warren J. Samuels, *Department of Economics, Michigan State University*

Research in the Sociology of Organizations
Edited by Samuel B. Bacharach, *Department of Organizational Behavior, New York State School of Industrial and Labor Relations, Cornell University*

Research in Transportation Economics
Edited by Theordore E. Keeler, *Department of Economics, University of California, Berkeley*

Research in Urban Economics
Edited by J. Vernon Henderson, *Department of Economics, Brown University*

Research on Technological Innovation, Management and Policy
Edited by Richard S. Rosenbloom, *Graduate School of Business Administration, Harvard University*

Monographs in Series

Contemporary Studies in Applied Behavioral Science
Series Editor: Louis A. Zurcher, *School of Social Work, University of Texas at Austin*

Contemporary Studies in Economics and Financial Analysis
Series Editors: Edward I. Altman and Ingo Walter, *Graduate School of Business Administration, New York University*

Contemporary Studies in Energy Analysis and Policy
Series Editor: Noel D. Uri, *Bureau of Economics; Federal Trade Commission*

Decision Research - A Series of Monographs
Edited by Howard Thomas, *Department of Business Administration, University of Illinois*

Handbook in Behavioral Economics
Edited by Stanley Kaish and Benny Gilad, *Department of Economics, Rutgers University*

Industrial Development and the Social Fabric
Edited by John P. McKay, *Department of History, University of Illinois*

Monographs in Organizational Behavior and Industrial Relations
Edited by Samuel B. Bacharach, *Department of Organizational Behavior, New York State School of Industrial and Labor Relations, Cornell University*

Political Economy and Public Policy
Edited by William Breit, *Department of Economics, Trinity University* and Kenneth G. Elzinga, *Department of Economics, University of Virginia*

Please inquire for detailed brochure on each series

 JAI PRESS INC., P.O. Box 1678
Greenwich, Connecticut 06836

Telephone: 203-661-7602   Cable Address: JAIPUBL